K.B. & Me

K.B. & Me:

The Tale of a Cancer-Fighting Rabbit With an Attitude

Judith Trotter Short

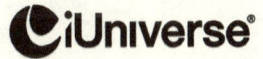

K.B. & ME:
THE TALE OF A CANCER-FIGHTING RABBIT WITH AN ATTITUDE

iUniverse books may be ordered through booksellers or by contacting:

iUniverse
1663 Liberty Drive
Bloomington, IN 47403
www.iuniverse.com
844-349-9409

ISBN: 978-0-5951-7092-0 (sc)
ISBN: 978-0-5957-2220-4 (e)

Print information available on the last page.

iUniverse rev. date: 08/21/2020

This book is dedicated to all the family, friends, business associates, doctors and nurses (as numerous and bright as the stars) for their care, love, prayers and support during the most difficult time of my life—and especially to my husband Roger, who made my vision of K.B. a reality.

Special thanks to Michael Lee, McKenrick Lee Photography, for the cover photo.

Contents

Chapter One

"Going to the Beauty Parlor"

I am so glad that I went to the "beauty parlor" or I wouldn't have been home to take the phone call telling me that I had flunked my mammogram.

You see, around our house, going to the "beauty parlor" (a term which is amusing in itself with its somewhat archaic quality) is a euphemism for going to the dentist. I have a genuine phobia about that, not based on any unreasonable fears, but on a lifetime experience of abuse at the hands of those in the dental profession.

This "beauty parlor" nonsense all got started when our friend Linda was going to have some major dental work done. When she told us, she started going into way more detail than I wanted to hear, so I sat with my fingers in my ears doing that "La, la, la, I'm not hearing this" routine.

A short time later she asked my husband, Roger, and I if we could give her a ride to the "beauty parlor." Somehow Rog got this all mixed up and thought she was going to the dentist and just didn't want to use the "D" word in front of me. So he volunteered to give her a ride and (lo and behold!) she was actually getting her hair done. So after that, the term just sort of stuck.

The saga of how my "beautician" figured into all this began one morning when Rog couldn't get me out of bed. Since we normally get up at 4:30 a.m. to go to the fitness center, this was unusual. (Yeah, I know that is a sick time to work out, but it is the only way to work it into our schedules. Evening workouts are just too easy to blow off.)

So Roger went off to work and called later to check on me. "What's wrong?" he asked.

"Uh," I wavered. *OK, how could I not tell him?* "Well, I, uh, I have a toothache."

"How long has this been going on?" was his next question in a most suspicious tone.

I paused so long that he asked if I was still there.

"Since Father's Day weekend?" I finally squeaked out.

He exploded. "You've had a toothache since June?" (This was now late August.)

"Well, yeah, but up until now the ibuprofen seemed to be taking care of it." Now this was starting to hurt worse than my tooth.

"Why didn't you say anything about it?" He was incredulous.

The answer seemed pretty obvious to me. "Because I knew you'd make me go to a, you know, 'beautician.'"

Which is, of course, exactly what he did.

He even called our friend Angie who serves our breakfast every morning at the Village Kitchen to get the name of her dentist. She had confessed to being a dental coward too and just had some major work done. She had raved about how great (and relatively painless) this guy was.

So I sat by the phone and cried for an hour trying to get up the nerve to place the call to even get an appointment.

I have no idea what Jackie, the receptionist, thought when she took my call that day. I started blubbering like a complete idiot. I wouldn't have been surprised if she'd hung up on me, then taken the phone off the hook to keep an insane person like me far, far away from Dr. Brennecke's office. If I had encountered someone like me I'd probably have gone so far as to get the phone number changed! But she was most patient and that was the first indication of what a first-rate "beautician" I had found. *Anyone smart enough to hire this woman must not be too bad,* I was thinking.

Here I had put off going to the "beautician" for five years and I was going the very next morning. Since I don't believe that there's any such thing as a coincidence, it has to be cosmic, the part that the "beautician" played in all this!

So this wonderful man gave me Novocaine (so much that my ear was even numb for hours), nitrous oxide and a prescription for pain pills. I dearly love my husband of 20+years so don't misunderstand when I say that all I could think of was, *Where has this man been all my life?*

"So, what did you do?" I asked him as I was getting out of the chair.

"Well," he said and it seemed that he was trying really hard not to grin, "that was about the first half of a root canal."

I was stunned. This guy was more than good!

He warned me that my mouth would be pretty sore once the numbness wore off. (And he was correct.) But that's what the prescription was for, right?

So I went home, took a pain pill and went to bed.

I think I was still asleep when the phone rang.

*   *   *

Three hours later and after I let my pain pill wear off I was driving to the Barrett Cancer Center. I was numb, in shock. This couldn't be happening.

You have to come in right away; we've got you squeezed in to see Dr. Hasselgren, one of the breast surgeons. I was about to meet my second wonderful man du jour.

This kind but authoritative man with a touch of an accent explained that I had not only flunked my mammogram, I had flunked it big time. Besides the fibroidy mass my doctor and I had felt on top of my left breast for the past year, there was also a small lump in the bottom half of the same breast.

"I am very concerned," he said pointedly and more than once.

Fear started setting in. This had to be some kind of drug-induced nightmare brought on by my morning's visit to the "beautician." I felt detached, like I was watching a movie about someone else.

Dr. Hasselgren recommended a biopsy of both areas but would first do something called a needle aspiration where he would remove a few cells with a needle right then and there. These would be sent to a lab but he warned me that this test was inconclusive and no matter what it showed, he would still recommend that I have the biopsies done in a few weeks.

Now, about this needle aspiration…Can we just say that this puts a root canal in a whole different perspective? The nurses were so understanding, when I had a hard time trying to answer their questions. I explained that I had just had the first half of a root canal that morning.

"Oh, you poor thing!" they exclaimed. I figured it also had them thinking that this put their worst day into perspective too.

Dr. Hasselgren came back in with a needle I can't even describe and one of these aforementioned compassionate nurses. "You can hold my hand when he inserts the needle," she told me, "because this is definitely going to hurt."

"Oh, I'll be OK," I told her. *I've really never had a problem with needles or shots, I'm a big girl,* I thought.

She reached over and took my hand anyway.

I just hope it wasn't the one she writes with.

*   *   *

This was on a Thursday and I left with an appointment for the following Tuesday when the test results would be back.

I went home and took another pain pill.

I just knew that telling Rog would be the hardest thing I'd ever done in my life. But it never occurred to me not to tell him right away. It would be pretty obvious anyway that something was up (since I was holding my jaw with one hand and my breast with the other!) This also wasn't a toothache that I could cover up for two months.

So we sat on the couch and held each other and cried.

Roger was wonderfully reassuring. "We're going to get through this together," he said holding me tightly. "Oh, I wish it were me instead of you…You just have to be OK; I just don't know what I'd do if I lost you."

I have absolutely no idea what we did that weekend. I do know that we did not breathe a word to anyone about any of this. I know that we talked to son Steve who lives in Atlanta with his wife Becky and our two adorable grandchildren, Spencer and Audrey. I also know that I talked to daughter Suzanne who lives in Cincinnati about our usual Monday night plans for dinner and laughing together through "Melrose Place."

But nothing was said about the news of the week.

On Tuesday Roger accompanied me to Dr. Hasselgren's office. How many days are there between Thursday and Tuesday that it could possibly seem like such a long time? All weekend long I had felt more helpless than afraid. The waiting and not knowing were the hardest parts. I went to work on Friday and Monday in a haze.

It was so important for Roger to be there with me. There was no way I could hear this news alone. And there was no way he wanted to wait somewhere for me to call him with the news. We both needed to hear it as soon as possible, and together. I was so proud of him and of his obvious love for me as he marched close behind me into the small examining room. *Most husbands would feel awkward and self-conscious in this situation,* I thought. But Roger was his usual optimistic self which gave me a great deal of strength. He was trying very hard to be strong for both of us.

Here's where selective listening kicks in:

Dr. Hasselgren entered the room, shuffling through my file. I introduced Roger to him and we all sat down. "The results of this test," he began, "show no cancer cells, but I am still very concerned."

Through the wonders of selective listening, Roger heard: "No cancer cells."

I heard: "I am still very concerned."

We left with an appointment for the biopsies to be performed in two weeks on Friday, September 5. Roger felt totally relieved. I felt somewhat on edge. The fat lady had not sung for me. I had a sense of dread that this wasn't over.

"This is such great news," I remember Roger saying. "I guess they still have to do the biopsies to be totally certain, but no cancer! This is just great."

I tried to temper his enthusiasm with realism. We're both involved in the construction industry: he as an architect; me as head of a construction trade association. Perhaps an illustration from real life would help him to understand that I was far from off the hook with this thing.

"It's sort of like soil borings," I began.

When a building is planned, engineers conduct soil borings on the site. They drill deep holes and take out samples of the soil to see if the area is suitable for building. Remember the Sunday school song about the wise man and the foolish man selecting their building sites on either rock or sand and the subsequent results? OK, so you get the picture.

"The problem with soil borings though," I continued in my illustration with Roger, "is that it all depends on where they drill the holes."

We had both known of instances, exceptions to the rule, where the soil borings showed solid ground, but when the excavation began, problems were unearthed, so to speak.

"Yeah, that's right," Roger nodded.

But he still didn't get it, or basically didn't want to. Selective listening again. Maybe the needle aspiration didn't show any cancer cells because it just didn't happen to *hit* any cancer cells. Maybe that was why Dr. Hasselgren kept saying, "I am very concerned."

That weekend we flew back east to visit friends in Washington and Baltimore where we had just lived for seven years. "Mum's the word," I warned Roger. I still didn't want anyone to know about any of this.

While we were there I did talk to my friend Victoria though because she had been through a similar scare a couple of years before, when we were neighbors. We talked about the biopsy procedures in general and about my fears.

"The needle biopsy didn't show any cancer cells, but what if there IS something there?" I asked her tearfully.

"But honey, Roger seems so sure that it's OK," she objected.

Then I told her about selective listening.

We hugged and she reassured me. And I didn't tell another soul.

The next weekend we flew to Atlanta to be with the kids and Roger started "outing" me the minute we walked in the door.

During the weekend, we talked about the biopsies openly but everyone generally adopted Roger's attitude of, "It's only a formality" or "They'll probably just take the lumps out."

Looking back, Becky told me that in an effort to stay positive, no one wanted to voice the terrible "what if" question. Innocent until proven guilty…Benign until proven otherwise. I think that was exactly how I felt too.

All that weekend my breast still hurt from the "soil borings."

Chapter Two

Those Three Little Words

The "beautician" played yet another critical role in all this. When I went back on September 3 to get the rest of my root canal, Sherry, a temp, was working with Dr. Brennecke while his regular assistant was off for a few days. It seems that Sherry also teaches some classes at The Wellness Community, an organization that offers support to people with cancer and to their families.

Without mentioning what I was going through, Sherry, Dr. Brennecke and I had a really interesting conversation about healing, alternative medicine, and various authors or experts on the subject. We talked about instances that we either knew about or had heard about where "mind over matter" ruled.

Dr. Brennecke related how Sherry had used the relaxation techniques she taught at The Wellness Community to rid him of an excruciating headache the day before.

I shared with them Roger's often-repeated story of cutting his finger in shop class when he was in high school. Evidently, he had an "A" grade going in the class and was afraid that if the teacher saw that he had been careless it would affect his grade. He said that he cut his finger to the bone and willed himself not to bleed—and he didn't.

No such discussion can go anywhere without Bernie Siegel's name coming up. The author of *Love, Medicine and Miracles,* Bernie is a doctor who explores the attitudes of his patients who seem to get better, or at least live longer with a higher quality of life. He compares these to patients with attitudes that seem to rush toward death. Rog and I read the book about ten years before this and had given copies of it to several friends with cancer.

*   *   *

So I was elated when Sherry said, "Did you know Bernie is going to be speaking here in Cincinnati on Monday night?"

No, I didn't know and I wouldn't have known and I would have missed it. This was on a Wednesday. I had the biopsies on Friday, two days later.

Roger and I arrived at University Hospital and rode up in the elevator to the Same Day Surgery Center. I had been there earlier in the week for pre-admission testing and had scoped it out. It looked like Roger would have a comfortable place to wait at least.

Plus, every staff person we encountered—from doctors and nurses to aides who wheeled you from place to place—treated us with such concern as human beings, not just as parts on an assembly line in their "factory" job that happened to be in a hospital. This was my first clue that current health care providers have discovered that patients are customers who have a choice about where they receive their care. I was impressed.

They took us into a holding room where various nurses came and went. Roger and I held hands and smiled at each other.

For three weeks I had noticed items every day in the newspaper about cancer in general or about breast cancer specifically. I had a sense of foreboding each time I saw an item, but didn't say anything. Never before had I seen so much about the subject. Was Someone trying to tell me something, prepare me for what was to come? Again, I don't believe in coincidences.

Roger maintained his upbeat, Pollyanna attitude the whole time. We were just going to get this over with and nothing was going to happen to my beautiful breasts. I would have a couple of small incisions for the biopsies and our friend Victoria had assured us that these wouldn't leave long-lasting scars. Everything was going to be just fine.

I would be receiving a local anesthetic with an IV backup—which meant that I wouldn't be knocked out, but I pretty much wouldn't remember anything either. This is supposedly much easier on your system to recover from than the general anesthesia used for most surgeries. The process would take about two to three hours. I wasn't frightened by the experience although my exposure to hospitals for my own use hadn't gone much beyond having my tonsils removed when I was in the second grade. I just wanted to get this over with and find out exactly what was going on inside me.

When I returned to the holding area after the surgery, Roger didn't appear right away. When he did, he seemed a little weepy.

"I wasn't going to do this," he apologized, hastily wiping away tears. Then he went on. "I just talked to Dr. Hasselgren. He, uh, he said it didn't look good, but he won't know for sure until the lab does the pathology report. He'll call us tonight." Then he kissed me, and held my hand very tightly.

Again, I felt numb. Dopey from the procedure, yes, but in shock as well. My conscious mind would not admit that the fat lady was warming up in the wings. This had to be a mistake. This had to be a nightmare that I would wake up from. I could not possibly have anything seriously wrong with me. I couldn't even think of, much less pronounce, the "C" word aloud.

I learned later that Dr. Hasselgren had found Roger in the waiting area following the surgery and had taken him into a private room with comfortable chairs and a phone. He wanted to prepare Roger for the news he was sure would follow. The man is a professor of surgery at the University of Cincinnati and he had performed enough of these procedures to know what he was looking at. This wonderful man who had kept saying that he was very concerned had his suspicions confirmed.

Roger used the phone to call the kids, Victoria, and our friend Dazy in Baltimore.

"You called Dazy?" I exclaimed. "But she didn't even know anything was going on!"

I figured that in his rattled state, he either forgot who knew or figured that everyone would know very soon anyway. (Actually, he didn't have Victoria's new work number and called Dazy to get it.) Confusion reigned.

At about 6:30 that night, Dr. Hasselgren called with the pathology report. Roger and I got on two phones so we could both talk to him. It doesn't become real until you hear your doctor say those three little words that you don't believe you will ever hear: "It was cancer."

As he reviewed my options, he kept calmly repeating, "'This is not the end of the world."

But as far as I could see, it was the end of mine. I hung up the phone, threw myself on the couch and burst into loud, soul-wrenching sobs.

*   *   *

That was the worst night for Roger, me, and probably anyone who receives that kind of news. Flashes came back later, one at a time, of my initial reactions: agony at the thought of losing my breast; anger that this had happened to me; fear of leaving my loved ones before I wanted to; helplessness at not being in control; and disbelief that this was happening at all. All these and probably more emotions washed through me, one on top of the other, like a great dam had burst. By the time I fell asleep, I felt that I had confronted the demons and cast them out.

Roger kept reassuring me of his love no matter what happened to my breast and that all he really cared about was not losing me. I had an ice pack across my chest to alleviate the soreness from the biopsies, but he held me tenderly, kissing my hair and my eyes, and let me cry, trying bravely not to cry with me.

The next day I was ready to confront this thing. For many people acceptance is the hardest part, and many people spend a long, long time in that state. I don't recommend it, because you have too much to do and too many major decisions to make in a short period of time.

We spent a lot of time on the phone, calling family and friends. Now that it was a certainty, I wanted to call on my entire support system. I needed their love, their strength, their positive thoughts and prayers.

Roger went out and bought about $200 worth of books and meditation tapes. We both read a lot. I wanted to know more about what I was facing. I wanted to be able to ask intelligent questions. I wanted to be able to read and comprehend the pathology report when I got my hands on it. I wanted to make intelligent, not emotional, decisions about what kind of treatment I would or would not receive.

*   *   *

I was shocked to read the statistics: 185,000 women are diagnosed with breast cancer every year and 44,000 die from it every year! Breast cancer will hit one woman out of every eight. One in eight! If I were at a party with seven other women, I would never even win the door prize! Yet somehow, I had won this one! Me! The healthy one. The one who watched my weight and went to the fitness center at the crack of dawn! The one with no history of cancer in my family, on either side, breast or otherwise.

Cancer is the great equalizer. It doesn't play by the rules. Besides these shocking numbers on breast cancer, more than one million

Americans are diagnosed with cancer every year. Plus eight million either have a history of cancer or are currently undergoing treatment!

At about the same time that all of this was happening to me, two men that were business associates of mine were diagnosed with different types of cancer. What was up with this epidemic that had suddenly invaded my world?

Breast cancer stories came out of the woodwork—from every friend or business associate I talked with. These were encouraging stories of a wife, a mother, a sister or an aunt—who had been through breast cancer five, ten or twenty years before. OK, so I was one of eight. I was immediately determined to be one of those who lives to tell the story.

I wasn't just going to be a cancer "survivor" either. I really don't like that term. For me, it carries negative connotations of someone who has been through a major disaster where no one is expected to come out alive, but miraculously someone does. Just by chance.

I wasn't going to take any chances. I made up my mind to face this head on, learn as much as I could, laugh as much as I could, and maintain a positive attitude no matter what.

The following Monday I was shaking Bernie Siegel's hand.

I took our old, somewhat battered copy of his book and he signed it for me. As he shook my hand he looked me in the eye and said, "Why are you here tonight, Judy?" And I told him.

He said something to me then that I will never forget. He even used it in his talk later. He told the crowd in the convention center, "I met a woman here tonight who was just diagnosed with cancer on Friday. I told her she's going to do all right because she's way ahead of the game. She's here tonight, and she's facing this and dealing with her cancer already. Most people would still be in denial."

I knew that Bernie was right. I would do whatever it might take to continue staying ahead of the game. And that's exactly what I've done.

I also said a prayer of thanks for my "beautician."

My support system was firmly in place and growing. Our friend Darla drove and took us to hear Bernie Siegel that night. As a brave and steadfast friend, she was also a wealth of knowledge. I knew that she had learned it the hard way when her husband, our friend David, had died of cancer two years earlier. The four of us had been friends for so many years and had known such fun times. I knew that it wasn't easy for Darla to be back in the midst of another cancer battle.

Darla could provide practical information as well as emotional support. She knew about the importance of getting flu and pneumonia shots. She mentioned the value of washing your hands several times a day since most germs are passed that way. With a depleted immune system, simple things like this and staying away from people with the sniffles becomes vital. She could also tell us that the rollercoaster of emotions was typical.

We had already discovered that one day we could be on an "I can do this" high followed the next day with a "This cannot be happening" low. I alternated between rage that this was happening and disbelief that it was happening to me. I felt caught up in love for all my friends and family, alternating with hate for this disease and the "stupid" researchers who can't seem to figure out what causes it! Roger and I would experience a positive high, followed by tears and depression. We both had these highs and lows, usually at the same time, but not always.

I'm not all that keen on rollercoasters anyway as an adult. As a kid I had loved them but back then I never thought of them breaking down. When you're young, you just jump on board and go for the thrill. Maybe that makes it a perfect analogy for emotions. Maybe the secret to survival is to just let go and ride it out. But you can control whether you enjoy the ride or have your eyes closed in terror the whole time. I decided it was time to bring back that youthful enjoyment of a thrilling ride and not let the negative "what ifs" cloud my thinking.

I don't want to sound like some positive thinking "nut" or paint an endlessly rosy picture. You will still have days that you wake up and think, *I just had a really horrible nightmare.*

Then the reality of those three little words, "It was cancer," hits you anew. And you know it's not a bad dream after all.

While not in denial, I had these same thoughts. *How could I have cancer? I'm not sick!*

The very possibility of my death frightened Roger more than it did me. I don't think that I have ever had a true fear of death—a fear of a nursing home is higher on my list. I've always thought of death as just a new experience, another dimension. But I did have fears about leaving others behind, especially Roger. There were just so many things I had to do and those thoughts filled me with such great sadness: getting to see the grandkids grow up; places not yet traveled to; major plans for growth and expansion I had launched at work.

One of the most startling facts I learned in my "Crash Course on Cancer 101" was that breast cancer takes a long time in making its presence known. All it takes is one little cell to go haywire, then others follow suit. But a tumor or mass large enough either to be felt as a lump in the breast or show up on a mammogram, has been growing for nine to ten years!

So why wasn't there some blood test or something to detect it five years ago, before it got so large? I thought of all the things we had done in the past decade—major relocations, job changes, marriages of our children, the birth of grandchildren. And all this time, this terrible thing had been growing inside me without my knowledge! I had thought I was pretty health conscious, but all this time I hadn't been conscious of this ticking time bomb.

Chapter Three

Enter K.B.— the Bunny with a 'Tude

Everyone wants to meet K.B., if they haven't already. He's my Killer Bunny. He's my visualization aid to help me fight cancer. In all the books I read in that short period of time, I learned that many cancer patients use visualization techniques to call on their bodies' own healing power. In one instance, a woman visualized that her white cells were polar bears, clawing out the cancer cells and eating them. Another used white sharks.

I thought those were WAY too violent. I don't even like to see those critters in movies!

So I told Rog I was going to use bunnies. My white cells would be white killer bunnies, hopping and munching, hopping and munching, ridding my body of these hideous cancer cells. They would be ferocious, but I could trust them not to turn on me. They were rabbits with an attitude. They were cancer-fighting rabbits. AND—since they WERE rabbits—they would reproduce quickly—which is what you want your white cells to do, to help build the body's immune system.

After a few days I could tell something was bothering Roger. I thought we were over the glum, brooding, depressing part and were taking a positive approach.

"Honey, you seem really down," I finally ventured. "What's wrong?"

17

He thought about it before answering, "It's this bunny thing of yours. It's just too passive. I'm afraid you're not fighting hard enough, that you're going to give up like your dad did."

My father had suffered a stroke more than fifteen years before. From the first day he seemed to accept his coming death as a certainty, although it was six months before he passed away. No matter how much we encouraged him and urged him to try, to fight, he just gave up. I could understand how Roger might think that such a tendency could be hereditary.

"But it's not passive," I explained. "These are KILLER bunnies! They're ferocious and determined. They have scary, spiky teeth. They have a mission!"

Then I drew him pictures of them.

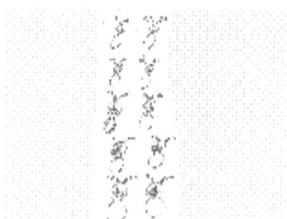

When he looked at my crude sketches of K.B. and his friends, all Roger said at first was "Oh," with just a touch of wonder in his voice.

Then he looked at me in amazement and the worry seemed to melt off his face. "These ARE Killer Bunnies."

Well, thank heavens he got it and realized that I was, indeed, fighting this.

So before I entered the hospital for my next round of surgery, he drove all over the city trying to find a white plush rabbit. Do you have any idea how difficult that is eight months before Easter? He could find bears, cats and every other animal on the planet. He went doggedly (pardon the pun) from store to store until he finally found the only white plush rabbit in all of Greater Cincinnati. Then, because it was a month before Halloween, he found some scary plastic monster teeth and super-glued them over the bunny's mouth. The teeth even glow in the dark. And K.B., my Killer Bunny, was born.

I placed K.B. where I could see him every day. Every moment I looked at him was a reminder that my body had to get to work, fighting off these cancer cells. From what I had read, cancer cells get out of hand when there are just too many of them for your immune system to battle effectively. I believed that empowering my immune system to fight harder would assist the doctors and the medicines to do their jobs. I was determined to take control.

K. B. went to the hospital with me. He either sat on the foot of the bed looking at me, or up on top of the TV where I could always see him. Every visitor to my room got the full explanation of who he was and what he was doing there.

One doctor was surprised that I knew about white cells. I told him that I had been reading a lot. It perplexed me to learn that it was unusual for a patient to have knowledge of his or her own disease. In a battle with any disease, but especially a life-threatening one like cancer, I think it is vitally important for the patient to ask questions, read books, talk to people who may have had the same disease or treatment. It is important to understand what the medical professionals are doing and why, what the medications or treatments are supposed to do, how they work, what their side-effects are. In other words, the patient cannot and should not be passive. It is YOUR disease so you have to get involved with it!

None of my doctors or nurses were ever put off or threatened when I asked questions either. If they had been, I was prepared to be confrontational if I had to. I would not be patronized or ignored, but fortunately was never made to feel that way.

All the doctors and nurses got a big kick out of K.B. A nurse came into my room one day, though she wasn't even assigned to me. She looked around at all my flowers then spotted K.B.

I started to explain but she interrupted me and said, "There he is! Oh, I've heard all about him." It must have been quite the buzz around the nurses' station about the wacky woman down the hall with the scary rabbit!

K.B. went to chemo with me too and sat where he could watch the drugs going in. The idea was for the chemo to create a famine and make K.B. and his friends starve and have to forage for food. Then they would search out and find the cancer cells and eat them. That would make them stronger. And well, they are rabbits…so then they would multiply! And multiply was exactly what I wanted my white cells to do!

All the nurses at the oncologist's office insisted on taking him around to show him to everyone there, including other patients. I always secretly hoped that some of those other patients would be inspired by him. Each time I went for a chemo treatment, the staff would greet him saying, "Hi, K.B.!" Or, "The Killer Bunny is back!"

One young nurse smiled one day when I explained K.B. and said, "Wow, that's really great! Where did you hear about doing that?"

No one had ever asked that before and I had to pause before answering, "I just made him up."

*   *   *

I took K.B. to my support group at The Wellness Community to meet everyone there as well. Weeks later several of the women said that they had told everyone they knew about him. His reputation was constantly growing.

Many times when friends and family sent gifts they would include a note saying, "This is something to help you and K.B. fight those cancer cells." or "How are you and K.B. doing?"

When Victoria, Dazy and our friend Bambi came to visit from D.C. one weekend after I got out of the hospital, they couldn't wait to see him. All weekend long, we would keep him with us whatever room we were in.

In the morning Dazy would walk in the living room, spot him and say, "Good morning, K.B."

At one point Bambi picked him up and put him in her lap, facing her. She made snarly faces back at him, then sat him back in his corner of the couch.

During the middle of one conversation Victoria simply burst out laughing. "K.B., you are cracking me up with your little pink feet and pink nose and that ferocious face."

The same thing would happen when Darla, our friends Linda and her husband Rick, or any other friends dropped by.

K.B. had become an accepted part of our social circle.

I always tried to be careful when I carried him out in public so that his face was turned toward me. I didn't want to give any small children nightmares, for crying out loud!

I kept him where I could see him every day. At home, I would move him from room to room to keep him with me, wherever I was. He still makes me smile when I look at him. Sometimes I would bare my teeth and snarl back at him, "GRRRRR! Go sic 'em, K.B.!"

Now when people ask me how I came up with K.B., I have to honestly tell them that I do not know. He just came to me, my own creation. When Roger presented him to me in his physical form, he looked just like my crude drawings and just as I had envisioned him. Plus Roger made sure I didn't see him until he was "complete" with his scary teeth in place. So I never saw him and have never thought of him as a cute, cuddly child's toy.

Roger and I have always (it seems) been into visualization. It probably goes back to the 1970's when we first read the book *Mind Games*. That phase undoubtedly worked better for Roger than for me, since I did most of the reading. He claims I have a wonderful voice. At any rate, it enabled him to sleep during periods of insomnia.

Prior to this, our method had been for me to tell him boring stories of my childhood, growing up on a farm in Indiana. He would get sleepy and say, "Tell me about dressing up your cat in doll clothes." I actually did this and it was a lot of fun (for me, not necessarily for the cat). However, it did somewhat disturb me that he thought these scintillating stories were sleep-inducing. Our grandson Spencer is enthralled with them.

After reading the *Mind Games* book, we would use our own personal calming scenes to lessen stress. To this day, Roger will envision himself "taking a little trip to the Bahamas" when he is under stress. He envisions that he is on a tranquil beach with all the accompanying relaxing images, smells and sounds.

We both have used these techniques to accomplish our own satisfactory results in business situations. Before going into a sales meeting or what could be a confrontational situation, we envision what the END of the meeting will be like according to our own scripts. Everyone is relaxed and smiling, asking meaningful questions. We answer with confidence, smiling and calm as well. The meeting would end with everyone shaking hands around the table, and us closing the deal, solving the problem or whatever. When the real meeting concluded, we would find that our vision of the happy ending was most often exactly what happened.

A few years later we encountered this same approach in videotapes aimed at improving one's skill in given sports, specifically golf or tennis. The idea was that you would watch these tapes where experts delivered the perfect performance. As you watched, you would envision that it was YOU making these amazing moves. Then, when in real life you were playing the sport, you would play back these mental tapes of you in these extraordinary (to us) performances. And most of the time, it was actually effective. We were at least moderately better than before.

So this whole concept of visualization was not foreign to us. It might sound freaky or weird to some. But I assure you that it is not. By planting the positive seeds of what you want the outcome to be, I do believe that you can positively influence that outcome.

For me to bring K.B. into my battle with cancer was the next extension of positive thinking methods I had been using for years. I encourage anyone with cancer to use such visualization techniques. These are helpful for fighting the disease, for controlling pain or nausea, for relaxation and sleep. Is it necessary to have an actual visual aid like K.B.? Not really. I just know that it helped me to have him around. To skeptics I would say, "What have you got to lose?"

Over time, it might be easy to forget to meditate or use visualization techniques. Schedules get busy or perhaps you don't feel well. Having a constant physical reminder helped remind me to stay an active part of my own battle.

Having an open mind in dealing with disease can have a positive impact as well. Your own past religious beliefs may be strengthened or expanded. You may find that you become a more spiritual person—which is significantly different from being "religious." Deeper awareness and sensitivity to your own feelings, your relationships with others and even how you react to casual acquaintances are not uncommon.

Roger commented one day after the three of us had been to the oncologist's office, "I think it's great that you're never embarrassed to carry K.B. around. A lot of people, including me, would probably be self-conscious walking into a doctor's office with a stuffed rabbit."

I smiled. "It would never occur to me. K.B. just belonged there as much as I did."

He is one tough bunny, but he had become a special friend as well.

Chapter Four

Be Careful What You Wish For

Whatever type of cancer a person has, there are always treatment options, and the patient should be the one to do the choosing. Medical professionals may strongly support or encourage certain options, but it is still up to the patient to decide what he or she wants to do. The patient has to ask pertinent questions to help make these decisions. What are the advantages or disadvantages of certain types of treatment? What are the chances of recurrence using various options? What is involved in the administration of each option? How effective is each option believed to be?

In my case, Dr. Hasselgren carefully outlined two treatment options for dealing with the cancer itself. I could have a lumpectomy to remove the cancerous mass, then have six weeks of daily radiation treatments. The disadvantages of this treatment (besides the necessity of radiation) were that there was a chance that all of the cancer might not be removed and that my breast would be disfigured from the extensive surgery.

Or I could have a mastectomy.

I had always thought that if I were ever faced with this decision, I would do anything rather than have a mastectomy. In reality, my response was exactly the opposite. I wanted to get this cancer out of me. I wasn't particularly thrilled with the prospects of radiation either.

There would also have to be another incision made in my underarm area to remove lymph nodes for further testing if I chose the lumpectomy option.

Most books I had read about breast cancer said that for most women, the first reaction to a cancer diagnosis is, "Am I going to die?" That was actually my second question. My first was, "Am I going to lose my breast?" When I then hit the second question, I realized that thousands of women DO die from this, so who cares about a breast? Though I always thought mine were important to me, in the greater scheme of things they really have nothing to do with my personality or who I am as a person. I had always been proud of my 34-D chest, but then I recalled the difficulty of finding bras that fit right, or any clothes in general. That's probably why I've always felt genetically defective as a woman—I hate to shop. It was always such a discouraging, tiring feat— if clothes fit on top, they were baggy in the bottom—suits, dresses, pants, and jeans.

There were also options of breast reconstruction to consider. I could choose to have this done at the same time as the original surgery, or later.

To me, this also seemed like a no-brainer. Why go through major surgery twice? Plus there was something emotionally reassuring to know that I would wake up from surgery and would still have two breasts. Granted, one of them wouldn't be the original, but it would still be a breast. It's like preventative maintenance almost, where you have something fixed before you even discover it's broken.

After the first shock of the diagnosis, I never cried after that over what I thought of as a lump of fat. It was replaced with a different lump of my own fat, so I never had the shock of feeling disfigured or maimed as so many women before me had. Even those who have reconstruction months or years after surgery say that prospect helps them deal with what they view as a temporary situation. Some women choose not to have reconstruction at all. Again, it's all a matter of personal choice that should be yours to make. Fortunately, insurance companies have realized (or been forced by Congress to realize) that breast reconstruction after cancer surgery is not merely cosmetic.

Once I made my decisions Dr. Hasselgren referred me to Wonderful Man Number Three Who Is Not My Husband: Dr. Neale, an incredibly gifted plastic surgeon. When Roger and I met with him for the first time, I immediately knew that I was in good hands. After examining me, Dr. Neale said that I was a perfect candidate for a type of reconstruction called a tram flap. Using this method, two abdominal incisions are made in sort of an oval pattern. This skin is then transplanted or grafted over the breast area. Then fat tissue is tunneled up under the skin to be formed into the new breast.

After all the debate about the safety of breast implants, I rather liked this option. This would be my own body tissue, relocated, rather than something foreign introduced into my body. The saline implants used now are very safe, but I liked this option. Plus, it would mean that I would get a tummy-tuck out of this deal. Was there a Divine Fairness Scale somewhere that measured out that I was going through enough dealing with cancer—maybe I should be rewarded with a tummy tuck? *At least there was some positive side to all this!* I thought.

But it reminded me of that old warning: *Be careful what you wish for.* How many times in my life had I said, "I would give anything to have a flat stomach"? Well, now I would have one and I would be giving up my breast to get it.

During that first consultation with Dr. Neale, I asked, " Do you have any idea how many years I've worked out every day trying to get rid of this spare tire?"

He smiled wryly and said, "Then God was looking out for you, because I have a use for this now."

Dr. Neale was reassuring and professional in his manner, inspiring our confidence in his skill. In a very quiet way, he conveyed kindness and compassion. I felt like I was going to have the Dynamic Duo operating on me: Dr. Hasselgren would remove the cancerous tissue and lymph nodes, then step aside while Dr. Neale put it all back together again. Roger always said he hesitated to shake hands with either one of them, feeling that they should take extra good care of those hands!

One of the other things that impressed me about Dr. Neale was that one of his nurses, Theresa, had the same breast cancer diagnosis, surgery and reconstruction two years before. He had a walking recommendation right there. How helpful it was to have someone there I could ask questions—who had actually been through it and could answer based on first hand knowledge and experience!

On two occasions Dr. Neale took a purple magic marker and drew marks where he would be making the incisions. At first I felt pretty ridiculous. As I lay on the table, I warned, "You better not be drawing a happy face on there!"

The second time he did his creative artwork was the day before surgery. He told me to be careful not to wash it off.

He then took photos that had something to do with insurance filings and my case history. "Can I get an 8" x 10" and some wallet size ones?" I joked.

I'm not sure that he always appreciated my flippant sense of humor. I was to discover later that he had his own wry sense of humor that I appreciated a great deal.

Dr. Neale's artwork actually gave me something of a relief when I checked into the hospital the next day. Since everything was clearly marked, there was no danger of them operating on the wrong side!

When I had the surgery Carol and Larry, two very dear friends who had recently retired to Arizona, came back to be with us and were absolute godsends. Larry was a physician and provided all I felt I needed in a second opinion. Dr. Hasselgren had even called him long distance to review my pathology report from the biopsies. It was comforting to have a friend reiterate information to make sure I understood everything and to be on hand in case there were any last-minute questions, changes or new discoveries. Carol was a nurse, so between the two of them I knew they'd look after Roger for me and provide the emotional support and love we both needed. I was worried that Roger would forget little things, like eating, which could play havoc with his diabetes.

Thoughts like this made me all the more determined to win over this disease. I had to take care of Roger, make sure he took his medicine and ate right. I had to be around to find all the things he's constantly losing—checkbook, keys, electronic organizer. I had to be around to love him and so that he could love me.

So the Three Musketeers (Roger, Carol and Larry) took me to University Hospital at the crack of dawn on the day I was to have surgery. I would be in the operating room for five to six hours and would be staying in the hospital for four to five days. K.B. went too. We made him stay in the car until after I had been moved to my room and he didn't seem to mind. I knew he could do his job from out there and it reassured me to know that he was near. He was my secret weapon.

*   *   *

I went into the surgery totally confident in my doctors and without fear. I wanted to get this over with. In fact, I remember joking and talking with the various doctors, nurses and attendants right up until the drugs started making me feel dopey. I kept telling myself that K.B. was at work and that I was going to wake up feeling great, maybe even a little hungry and thirsty. I felt at peace knowing that very soon this cancer would be gone.

I went into surgery around 7:30 a.m. and was wheeled to my room, fairly alert, around 2:30 that afternoon. I felt great, but thirsty, and insisted that the nurse get approval for me to have ice chips at once. My lips were dry and felt like they were cracking, so I asked her to find my lipstick. It felt so soothing when I put some on!

I sneaked a peek at my bandages and actually smiled. *OK,* I thought, *the bad part is gone and I'm going to look like I still have two breasts.* Even with the bandages, I could tell that the roll of fat around my middle that I had cursed for years was gone too. Well, relocated at least. I felt like a miracle had transpired. I didn't just feel great—I felt exuberant.

When Roger, Carol and Larry came in, they were amazed. I was back in the room a lot sooner than they had been led to believe that I would be. They were also stunned by my appearance.

"You're awake already!"

"You look great!"

"You're wearing lipstick?"

K.B. sat snarling at the foot of the bed.

I felt terrific. Granted, I had some heavy-duty drugs working. "The morphine pump is my friend" became an oft-quoted mantra.

Then the parade began. Since this was a teaching hospital, Drs. Hasselgren and Neale were always accompanied by an entourage of interns. They seemed to enjoy meeting K.B. too. Each time they came in the room they would look around to see where he was.

I looked so vital and alert that at 5:00 p.m. Dr. Hasselgren got me confused at first with a patient he had operated on the day before. "Have they gotten you out of bed yet?" he asked.

"No; it's kind of soon, isn't it?" I asked, thinking they were really rushing me.

"Oh, no, they usually get the patients up after 36 hours," he said looking at my chart. Then he glanced sharply up at me. "Wait a minute, Mrs. Short. We just operated on you this morning, didn't we?"

I felt like saying "duh" but didn't.

He just shook his head. " You do not look like someone who just came out of surgery a few hours ago."

I didn't feel like one either. I also thought it wasn't just the effect of the drugs. I felt happy and loved and confident. I felt in control. I felt that I HAD cancer when I checked into the hospital, but now I didn't!

After the parade that first day the flower cart crashed in my room. Well, not literally, it just looked like it. We were running out of space for the nearly 30 flower baskets I received. This outpouring of love made me feel like a queen, a celebrity. I held each one and marveled that all these people cared so much about me. When I checked out on Saturday, I had Roger and the head nurse distribute many of them around the hospital to spread the cheer.

That was just one aspect of the decorating of my room. Besides having a gorgeous view of downtown Cincinnati, the room had a TV with VCR, refrigerator, loveseat, small table and chairs. I've been in fancy hotels that weren't this nice! Roger brought in a pink tablecloth and a tabletop fountain from home. He plugged in the fountain amidst all the flowers so this pleasant bubbling sound gave an even more peaceful atmosphere to the room.

One night one of the nurses came in and just stood still by my bed for a moment. She smiled and said, "I'm working a double shift and have a headache that's been nagging me all day. It seems like every time I walk in your room for just two minutes, with the fountain and the flowers, my headache gets better." She patted my hand, turned and went back to work. It seemed that my room was a healing place for others as well as for me.

I had really lucked out in getting such a beautiful room. But no matter what your surroundings, you can still make a hospital room your own. Dress it up; bring comforting things from home. Bring a pillow, afghan, photo or some favorite knickknack. Even if you're only there a couple of days, it will brighten your outlook immensely.

Roger stocked the fridge with wine, cheese and assorted munchies. I didn't join in, but the next day he, Carol and Larry were enjoying their refreshments at Happy Hour. It created such a normal, festive setting. This is what the four of us would be doing if we were at either one's home together. *How many people feel at home in a hospital room?* I wondered.

When Dr. Neale stopped in to check on me, they all felt like they'd gotten busted, although it wasn't actually against any rules. "Glass of wine?" Roger offered sheepishly.

Dr. Neale declined, almost hesitantly, after he glanced at the label and saw that it was, indeed, some mighty fine wine they were drinking.

All of these things plus the kind and caring staff combined to make my hospital stay a truly healing event. No one woke me in the middle of the night to give me medicine. There were no loud noises or racket in the hallway or coming from other rooms. There was soundproofing around the window so that when the rescue helicopter landed on the roof right above me, I never heard it. We would sometimes see flickering sunlight or headlights like a strobe as the blades rotated, and look up to see it pass by the window.

At every shift change I would write down the name of my nurse and the aide or student assisting her. It helped me to be able to call them by name over the next eight hours, and they seemed to respond positively as well, knowing that I had taken the time to learn their names. For patients who want to receive caring treatment from their health professionals, I would advise remembering to treat those workers with the compassion and respect that you want to receive.

Humor is an important part of healing and it has certainly been a vital part of mine. I particularly appreciated seeing it from my medical professionals. It was reassuring, and I believe it reinforced my immune system and my body's response to their treatments.

I learned more of Dr. Neale's sense of humor the following week. When I went to his office the week after surgery, hobbling, bent over in what Roger often called my "Groucho Marx position," Dr. Neale stood at the end of a long hallway watching me make my way to the examining room. He smiled and said, "OK, on your mark, get set, GO!" As if I'd be running any foot races any time soon!

Later when he started to remove the drainage tubes from my incisions, he cocked his head to one side and asked, "Do you remember that old song, *I Never Promised You a Rose Garden*?"

"Yes," I nodded, somewhat surprised. I recalled it being a country/western tune and he didn't strike me as being a C & W fan.

"Well," he said, taking a deep breath, "that's pretty much appropriate in this situation. When I pull these tubes out, it's really going to hurt, but just for a moment."

As he proceeded, he softly sang the song under his breath.

I smiled and winced and squeezed Roger's hand all at the same time.

Chapter Five

Score: K.B.—15
Cancer—0

While I was still in the hospital, I grew stronger each day and my spir-its soared as well. I was allowed to select my own meals and eat any-thing I wanted. Our friends Tom and Jackie had sent a creative "floral" arrangement made of delicious cookies—decorated to look like doc-tors and nurses. These I promptly scarfed down, with only a little help from visitors.

There was a sense of anticipation though. I needed to feel more sure of my victory. I needed to know that the Fat Lady had packed up and gone home. The final pathology report would be back on Thursday. During the surgery fifteen lymph nodes were removed from under my arm near the cancerous breast. The presence of cancer in these nodes would indicate how much the cancer had spread. The danger this pres-ents is that when cancer is in the lymph system, it can be carried throughout the body—to the liver, lungs, colon, or bones. When this happens, the cancer is said to have metastasized. It's frightening to think that your breast cancer can show up somewhere else in your body! *That just wouldn't be fair!* I thought angrily. I didn't feel sick anywhere, so it had to be alright. (Of course, my breast never felt "sick" either and look how it betrayed me!)

When the news came in, the doctors could hardly wait to tell me. All fifteen nodes were clear! The final analysis of the cancerous mass in my breast showed that it was almost three centimeters wide—a fairly large, fairly advanced tumor. The doctors all seemed amazed that, especially with a tumor that size, the cancer had not spread to the nodes at all. I had been prepared mentally for at least some node involvement. Others whom I had talked with usually had two to four nodes that showed cancer.

This was exciting news! Each team of doctors seemed jubilant. I was ecstatic. *Ha! Ha! Ha! You stupid cancer!* I thought. *You are outta here!*

"You look younger," Carol observed. "You look like ten years just fell away."

How could this happen? Was it a miracle? It seemed like it to me.

I knew that K.B. and a host of others had been hard at work during the past month.

There had literally been thousands of people praying for me and sending me positive thoughts. My family was spread from Cincinnati to Georgia to Indiana to Arkansas to Kentucky to Colorado to New Mexico to Illinois. Many close friends and neighbors here in Cincinnati were joined by those in Arizona, California, Louisiana, Maryland, Virginia, Washington, D.C., and even St. Thomas in the Virgin Islands—all thinking of me and praying for me.

On top of this I had been the national president of the National Association of Women in Construction and had attended their annual convention a few weeks before surgery. Many of this group's 7,000 members in over 200 chapters throughout the U.S. knew me and were praying for me.

During that convention I was able to spend time with my friend Carol from Connecticut—who had breast cancer nine years before. I called her my "Poster Girl" since she was such an inspiration to me. She

kept telling me that I would be all right too. We had always marveled
how two people who were so different in so many ways could be so
much alike. We had always had many of the same experiences and such
similar goals. My outcome would be positive just like hers, she assured
me. I knew from fifteen years of friendship that Carol was a wise and
perceptive woman, and was usually right. We smiled and hugged a lot
once the initial crying together was over.

The week I had surgery I had to cancel my attendance at another
national convention of the Associated General Contractors, an organization I had worked for in Washington, D.C. and am still affiliated with
through my job in Cincinnati. With more than 33,000 companies as
members and several thousand in attendance at that meeting, I knew
that many in that circle were praying for me as well.

My colleagues in Cincinnati included people from nearly 400 companies in Allied Construction Industries, our local construction association.

My affiliation with the Cincinnati Rotary Club (among the ten
largest in the *world*) had all of their members praying for me too. One
man I didn't even know all that well at the time even called and prayed
with me on the phone several times.

Two of my friends were on a tour of France while I was in the hospital. In every town they stopped, they went to church and prayed for me.

There was a ripple effect in this ever-widening circle of people—
around the world—who don't know me, but know my friends and family, and were praying for me. Roger was designing a church at the time
and that entire congregation was praying for me—without ever having
laid eyes on me. Many of his other church clients passed my name on to
countless prayer chains.

This went on and on, beyond my own vision or knowledge or awareness to the point that I will probably never fully know how many people
were praying and sending me their positive thoughts.

I do know this, though it is something I can never prove and that
skeptics would dismiss totally: I will always believe to the core of my

inner soul that K.B., with the help of these thousands of people, had an impact on that positive pathology report.

Those who doubt might question why the tumor didn't vanish entirely. It didn't need to. It was being dealt with surgically. Why waste a miracle on something that could be fixed?

This was demonstrated to me in the most unusual way when I again made a trip to the "beautician" a couple of weeks after surgery. The tube that had been down my throat for the many hours of surgery had pressed against the crown on my front tooth, loosening it. It came out shortly after I got to my hospital room, while I was sucking on ice chips. I was just thankful it had not come out during surgery or I might have swallowed it! I kept it glued on with dental adhesive until I could get it more permanently reattached.

Roger had canceled my dental appointment right before my surgery, explaining that I would have to postpone the bridgework I was planning and why. So Dr. Brennecke and his staff were aware of my cancer diagnosis and had even called to check on me and sent me a get-well card.

I've never had such a reception in a "beauty parlor." They were all so concerned and genuinely glad to see me. Dr. Brennecke and I had a long talk while he was gluing my tooth back on. He said he had been praying for me ever since he heard the news and that if it was OK with me, he would like to pray with me before I left his office.

He did and we both got a little teary. I was deeply touched.

Reflecting on all this, I was overwhelmed with love and thankfulness. For nearly a month, all these people—known to me and unknown to me—were praying for me, thinking about me, sending me their positive thoughts and energy. Some of these people I would call deeply religious. Some I would call spiritual. All I would call filled with love. They were a non-denominational, non-partisan, non-sectarian crowd.

I also kept two journals. Roger gave me the first one and in it I wrote my thoughts, observations and emotions during all this. This is great therapy for cancer patients and I highly recommend it. It is for no one else to read unless you choose to share it. It has quite a cathartic effect to get out all of these thoughts and feelings that you may be hesitant to voice to someone else. Some may think that they can't do this, that they are not writers, that writing is a chore.

Entries can be brief at first, like a daily diary of what you did and where you went. From this it can then grow to include more about your response to these experiences. How did you feel on the way to the hospital or doctor's office? How did you feel afterwards? How are your family and friends reacting to all of this? How is it affecting your work life, your family life, and your daily life? How has it impacted your priorities and what you want to accomplish with your life?

Each person's answers to these questions will be different and each are valid. In most of the books I've read, I have encountered emotions and reactions that are so different from my own. In some cases I thought, *Wow, glad I didn't feel like that!* Or *Hey, is something wrong with me? I never felt like that!* In some instances I thought, *Yeah, right on, me too.* This is the ultimate test of your life and there are no right or wrong answers or feelings. They are simply your own.

Knowing this, Darla had given me a journal as well. Since I didn't need two volumes (even though I can write a lot) I used that one to record the names of all the people who called, sent cards, or flowers, or gifts, or e-mails. Flipping through that gave me strength as well, seeing all those names, some more than once.

I put all my cards in a large salad bowl and was amazed at how quickly it filled up. I also kept it where I could see it every day. Once in a while I would sift through, re-reading the cards and the notes that people had written. Often something would stand out that I may have read when I received the card, but had taken on a stronger, deeper meaning over time. It was an inspiration to reflect on all these people, how far away some of them lived, and how their thoughts had traveled over the miles to me.

Remember that I had called on this support network. I didn't just sit and wait for them to find out about me. I mobilized friends to help me contact people. Roger made calls. I contacted key people in all these organizations and asked them to put me on as many prayer lists as they could. I was not shy; I was not going to try to hide the fact that I had cancer. I needed these people and I needed them to know that.

*   *   *

Many people, friends who were cancer survivors or "fighters" if you'll use my term, told me later that they wished they could have been as open as I was when they were going through their initial cancer diagnosis and treatment.

One woman in particular said that she just didn't want anyone she worked with to know and as a result only about three knew. There were nearly 100 of us in that office and yet she denied herself the power of our friendship.

Each person is different; some people are very private and simply cannot imagine sharing such personal information with anyone other than their immediate family. I understand. I'm glad I was able to go the more public route because it was such a boost to my attitude, and, I believe, to my healing process.

As a result, people responded to me differently when they would see me and ask how I was doing. The question, "How are you doing?" was usually accompanied with a quick, "You look great!" And I felt great. It made me smile when they seemed so surprised.

I went back to work just two weeks after the surgery by attending an annual black tie industry awards gala that I simply couldn't miss. As vice-president of the foundation sponsoring the dinner, I told Roger that I needed to be there even if he had to take me in a wheelchair. My reconstructive surgery had resulted in swelling, and had given me my distinctive bent, Groucho-Marx style of walking.

But I was determined.

No fancy dresses or suits in my closet would fit. So I reached in the back for a 20-year old, full-length caftan that could pass as a formal dress, with the addition of large rhinestone earrings. When I bought it in the 1970's, I think it was termed a hostess gown, a "wear-at-home" garment for entertaining. I always thought of it as a bathrobe. But somehow I made the transformation work.

I was able to hobble into the dinner on Roger's arm, without a wheel-chair. Nearly 700 people at the dinner were surprised and happy to see me. I felt stronger for being there. It was important to me to see all these business associates and it was equally important for them to see and know that I was recovering and not at death's door. The reports at my office the next day were that I looked elegant in a long, flowing gown.

I had also called on my body's own healing powers to fight off these cancer cells, to eradicate them, to outnumber them. I felt strong, like a soldier in a battle, determined to win and that positive attitude was evident to all who saw me. That positive pathology report on those lymph nodes was physical proof to me that I would win this fight.

K.B., my Killer Bunny, and his mighty legions were prevailing.

I will never believe that this was not so.

Chapter Six

The Second "C" Word—Chemo

Following surgery Dr. Hasselgren referred me to an oncologist to further study my pathology reports and determine what types of follow-up treatment would be recommended for me. (Adjuvant treatment is the fancy medical term used for this, and usually refers to chemotherapy, other drugs, or radiation.)

Counting my "beautician" Dr. Brennecke, my surgeon Dr. Hasselgren and my plastic surgeon Dr. Neale, I had met three wonderful men (who were not my husband). I was about to meet Wonder Woman Number One (Who Was Not Me)! Enter Dr. Elyse Lower. Drs. Hasselgren and Neale both recommended her highly. Carol and Larry both said she was the best in Greater Cincinnati. There had been several newspaper articles recently, quoting her extensively, noting her particular expertise in dealing with breast cancer.

For all of these reasons, it took a couple of weeks to get an appointment. That was a somewhat disheartening fact, just to think that there were that many of us in town at this time who needed to see her. When I finally got an appointment for 6:30 at night, I realized fully what hours this woman must be keeping to work in all the patients who needed to see her.

I was warned that when I had an appointment with her, Roger and I should take plenty of reading material because she usually ran late. These people were quick to explain that we wouldn't mind waiting when our turn came—she ran late because she spent as much time as necessary with each patient, answering all their questions and explaining all procedures and options with them.

I had seen her picture in the paper and passed her in the hallway at Dr. Hasselgren's office, but the first time Roger and I sat down with Dr. Lower we were blown away. This attractive, bouncy, smiling, upbeat woman swept into the examining room and said, "Finally! Everyone has been asking me if I've met Judy Short yet!"

Who was "everyone?" I wondered, and she never did elaborate. It did make me feel like a special patient though, if she had already been talking to people about me. (Or maybe they were warning her about the crazy woman with the scary rabbit, I don't know.)

The three of us spent over an hour together, just talking. She reviewed the pathology report on the cancer itself and on the lymph nodes, explaining what each finding meant and its implications for treatment.

She even went into future medical considerations. For instance, because my cancer was rated as hormone receptive, when I enter menopause I will not be able to receive estrogen replacement therapy—that could "feed" the cancer and cause it to grow.

My bone scan showed some probable arthritis, which Dr. Lower said should also be checked out eventually with my regular physician. A bone density test could show whether I was in the beginning stages of osteoporosis—which is also usually treated with hormones, again which I would not be able to receive. *OK, I'll deal with all that down the road too,* I thought.

"The results from your lymph nodes are really positive," Dr. Lower said exuberantly. "That's really encouraging! Fifteen nodes were removed and since they were all clear, that's a very good sign that the cancer hasn't spread."

It was reassuring to know that she was as happy about that report as I was.

"But how many lymph nodes are there? Is that enough?" was my nagging question.

She explained that there are hundreds of nodes in our lymph system, throughout our bodies, with 50-80 under each arm. She assured me that 12-20 was considered an adequate sampling because these are on the "front line" so to speak. It would be rare for cancer to get past these and skip on to others, farther from the breast.

"However," she said, with a little frown, "there is no guarantee that microscopic cancer cells have not escaped or spread and just are not detectable yet. That's why I recommend a program of chemotherapy, every three weeks for six months. If we do nothing, the chance of those microscopic cells being out there somewhere give you a 35—40% chance of a recurrence. With the chemo treatments, we can reduce that to a 10-15% chance of recurrence."

Then she pulled out a handout, explaining the chemo drugs she recommended for me, how they worked, what their possible side effects could be. This was the beginning of a large folder of information I was to receive from her, carefully explained by either her or her nurse assistant.

From what I could tell, this looked like "chemo lite." The drugs were not as intense as some because we were not attacking a specific area of cancer that was known to have spread.

I considered it more of a precaution, like getting a flu shot. Or like flushing the antifreeze out of your car at the beginning of winter, before you add new. Sure, it wasn't going to be a breeze, but I also remembered the first flu shots given 20 years ago that made you as sick as if you'd had the flu.

The odds were convincing. I've gotten drenched on days when there was only a 30% chance of rain, so lowering those odds to 10% was pretty attractive to me! On days with a prediction of only a 10% chance of rain, I don't even bother carrying an umbrella.

"With these chemo drugs, I don't expect that you will get very sick either," Dr. Lower assured me, again with another handout. "We now have some very effective anti-nausea drugs that you will be receiving as well."

"What about my hair?" I asked, pushing a thin wisp behind my ear.

"Most people don't lose their hair with these drugs. At least it doesn't tend to fall out in clumps all at once, but it may thin some," she replied.

"Mine is thin to start with," I said glumly. I figured this part could be a real nuisance. I didn't want to waste time worrying about my appearance. I had more important things to do, like fight cancer!

Dr. Lower nodded and wrote out a prescription for a "full cranial prosthesis." *This is a hoot!* I thought. It turns out that this is the medical term for a wig. Then it can either be submitted to your insurance company for reimbursement, or itemized with your medical expenses on your income taxes!

Leave it to the bureaucrats. If you just go buy a wig, it doesn't count. I figured I'd get the prescription filled, again as a precaution. If nothing happened to my hair, it could come in handy if I was just having a bad hair day.

"But I won't have to have radiation?" I wanted this confirmed. This was something I really wanted to avoid, with stories I had heard of burns and skin discoloration. (I've since learned that this treatment has been vastly improved as well, and if it had been recommended I would have done it anyway. These treatment methods change and are improved constantly, so those in the future will be spared even more of the negative side-effects.) But the thought of getting "zapped" every day for six weeks unnerved me more than the thought of drugs.

"No radiation," Dr. Lower shook her head. "That only works when there's a specific cancer mass or tumor involved or an area where there is question as to whether all the cancer has been removed or is inoperable. Since you had a mastectomy, there's basically nothing left to point at."

When all our questions were answered, we left with instructions to call the next day to schedule my first chemo treatment. It never occurred to me not to do it. Some people do choose not to have any of these follow-up treatments, so again the patient really is in charge. But for me, I wanted to decrease the odds of recurrence.

I felt strong; I could do this. My heart goes out to those who have a harder time with chemo, but it's got to be worth it. For now at least, it's all that medicine can offer. I thought of it in terms of going to the "beautician"—you have to do what you have to do.

Roger and I had read a lot of books about alternative treatments. Some of them made sense; some sounded downright kooky. We decided there were certain things we could accept and began on those.

This included a home-cooked, even healthier diet than we had before. We added vitamins, minerals, and herbal supplements considered to have anti-oxidant, cancer- fighting properties. We drank green tea instead of coffee in the morning. It still contained caffeine, but not as much as coffee. It was also thought to have cancer-fighting advantages. We had red clover tea (a recommendation from my "beautician") that was effective for fighting any nausea or queasiness.

I talked to many people who were taking other alternative remedies—in addition to the traditional treatments. My opinion is this: If you believe in it, it will have positive effects for you. I also figure it can't hurt. It may cost you a little extra because insurance companies never pay for vitamins, but if you can afford it and want to, I say go for it.

Orientals, Native-Americans and others used herbal remedies for thousands of years and still find them effective today. Personally, I think there's a lot to be said for ancient wisdom. I also figured that I would try any weapon I could tolerate—after all, this was war!

A word of warning though about those odds and percentages. You can worry yourself into a frenzy over anything that isn't 0% and the higher the number, the more depressed you can get. It's better to hear those numbers, then dismiss them. They can plant negative thoughts and inhibit your immune system from fighting back as hard as it can. Self-fulfilling prophecies can take hold with thoughts like, "Wow, I've only got a 30% chance of surviving this—I'm not going to make it!" Those who think like that probably won't make it.

I would also warn doctors NOT to give out predictions on how long a person has to live. They don't have a crystal ball and that can be self-fulfilling as well since I have heard of people dying on the day that their doctor predicted. Let's face it, we all should have our affairs in order, but planning a specific check-out time should be avoided.

*   *   *

Roger, K.B. and I went to Dr. Lower's office for my first chemo treatment on the afternoon of Halloween. *How appropriate,* I thought. I wasn't afraid though. I was curious. *What would this new experience be like?* I was determined that it wouldn't make me sick.

Dr. Lower was elated to meet K.B. for the first time. She held him and looked him right in his snarly teeth.

"He is wonderful!" she exclaimed, laughing. Shaking her head and smiling at us she said simply, "This is really good."

Every time we went back, she always talked to him and greeted him. He became quite a regular fixture around her office. In December she asked why he wasn't wearing a red ribbon or some festive decoration. I told her that he didn't go in for any frivolous stuff; he had serious work to do.

While the IV was being hooked up, I sat in a very comfortable reclining chair with Roger in one next to me, just to keep me company. We could talk, read, nap or watch TV during the couple of hours all this took.

K.B. sat in front of me where he could keep an eye on the drugs being administered. I figured he could start intimidating those cancer cells as the first drop went in. K.B.'s expression said that he meant business in a Clint Eastwood, "Make my day" kind of way.

Dr. Lower was right (not that I would ever doubt a word from this wise woman). I didn't get sick at all following the first few sessions. I felt a little achy and sleepless, side-effects from the anti-nausea drugs. These things I could control with pain pills or other medications, and after taking it easy over the weekend, I was ready for work on Monday!

I went back to Dr. Lower's office alone in two weeks just to have my blood count checked.

"Where's K.B.?" were Dr. Lower's first words to me.

"I gave him and Roger the day off," I told her laughing, "since we're not really doing any work here today."

"But something occurred to me last week that I should have asked you," I said, looking down at the blood report. (The nurse always gave me a copy to take with me). "What should my white count be today? I should have had a specific number for K.B. and I to concentrate on. I didn't think of it until later, but it might have helped."

She chuckled, looking down at her own copy of the report. "Well, K.B. must have read my mind and known the number I wanted because this is right where it should be. It has dropped some, which is expected, because that means the drugs are working. But then it should start coming back up in the next week before your next chemo treatment."

I went home and told K.B. to get to work on it. He did. The following Friday the count was headed back up.

What a rabbit.

Chapter Seven

Reach Out and Touch Everyone

For many people with cancer, the experience can be a lonely one. It need not be so. It wasn't for me because I took charge.

Two weeks before my surgery I visited The Wellness Community (TWC). I had heard about this organization from Sherry at the "beautician's" office and from my friend Darla. I decided to check it out for myself.

Their literature stated that "TWC provides free psychological and social support services for cancer patients and their families. TWC's program helps cancer patients focus on quality of life, reduce stress and regain control of their lives. Services include support groups, stress management sessions, education workshops and social events."

Sounded promising to me. I learned that there are 18 such organizations throughout the U.S. with more being formed, funded by corporations and private donations. I found a warm and caring trained professional staff, assisted by volunteers who had experienced cancer in their own lives.

I felt fortunate to discover that the local TWC had just started a support group for newly diagnosed breast cancer patients the week before and they immediately enrolled me in the group. There were eleven of us and we quickly formed what I knew would be life-long bonds.

Many people are hesitant to join such groups, afraid to discuss their feelings and fears with total strangers. Instead I found it comforting and educational to be able to talk about surgery, drugs, treatments, emotions and everything else related to the experience of having cancer with others who were going through the same thing.

Roger and I started referring to the group as my "Cancer Club." Somehow it sounded more normal (and amusing to some) than calling it a support group.

From my Cancer Club cohorts, I learned about wig-buying. Advice included:

"Go right away, before you even start to lose hair so they can match your style and color better."

"Take friends with you—it makes it more like a fun shopping trip!"

"Keep hats handy around the house in case you need to answer the door and haven't put your wig on yet."

I figured that if I didn't lose my hair this would still be helpful information to know.

We were able to talk openly about how we felt when we were diagnosed and how our families responded. We could share our fears and cry together. We also laughed together a lot. We could say things that others might have thought outrageous but somehow it was OK to say it in front of each other. We could express our anger at our disease, at doctors, at the lack of research, at our pain, at our treatments.

Basically, there was no subject that was taboo, nothing that we could not discuss together.

We talked about how our husbands were handling our ordeal and again I felt loved and lucky. Roger made me feel desirable at all times. He never was grossed out by anything (except perhaps my gnarly, newly-constructed navel, which I found rather disconcerting myself). He wanted to look at my incisions immediately and touched my new breast regularly. He loved my flatter stomach. When I first got home from the hospital, he helped me shower, held the drainage tubes,

washed my hair, put lotion on me. I had heard/read about strained relationships and even divorces following breast surgery, but Roger assured
me that his love was for ME, and that never changed.

It seems that the cancer ordeal is often hardest on the healthy spouse.
It is difficult to watch someone you love in pain. It is terrifying to realize
that you could lose this person who is the center of your world. Support
groups for family members and spouses abound. At least it's important
to find a friend or someone to talk to.

My conclusion was that for the most part, a strong relationship will
get stronger after cancer. A weak one may deteriorate further.

I also shared with the group one particular experience I had with
anger—only to find that two other women had similar experiences.

I was expecting a phone call from Carol and Larry one night shortly
after my diagnosis. I quickly grabbed the phone when it rang, only to be
greeted by a perky telemarketer selling something. "Good evening, Mrs.
Short. I'm calling you this evening with some wonderful news."

"Well," I snapped, "Unless you're calling to tell me that I DON'T have
breast cancer, I don't think so!" I slammed down the phone.

"Wow," Roger said later. "I think you may have over-reacted there a bit."

When I told this story to my Cancer Club though, we all laughed and
they understood.

*   *   *

It caused a few chuckles and raised eyebrows if friends heard Roger
ask, "Are you going to Cancer Club this week?"

Are you going where? their faces would ask.

I liked calling it that. It made it seem like any other organization I
might belong to. Others in the group called it our "Wig Club."

And of course I always went. The only sessions I missed were the first
week, before I discovered The Wellness Community and the week I was in

the hospital. Even then, Ursula, one of the other Cancer Club members, came to visit me at the hospital and a budding friendship was formed.

In every community there are organizations like this, sponsored by hospitals or other groups. There are even studies that show that support groups have a positive impact on cancer recovery rates, quality of life and longevity. A study released by researchers at Ohio State University in 1998 indicates that the stress and anxiety of having cancer may lower the body's immune system. Those in the study with the most anxiety about their condition also had the lowest white blood cell count. All the more reasons to reach out to lessen stress and increase coping skills.

It takes a commitment on the part of the patient, and sometimes on their family members, to get to such meetings on a regular basis, but I believe it is definitely worth it. There are even individual organizations for every type of cancer.

Perhaps I was more tuned into all of these opportunities because I was recovering from surgery during October—Breast Cancer Awareness Month. I couldn't turn on the TV or radio, or open a newspaper or magazine without seeing or hearing some announcement about breast cancer.

Lying on the sofa with the TV remote control, it almost got to be too much on some days. *Click*..."Today on Oprah...Breast Cancer Epidemic in America" *Click*..."This month on HBO: a special look into the causes of breast cancer." *Click*..."Every day on Rosie O'Donnell, a spotlight on breast cancer." *Click*..."Lifetime TV features a special presentation on one woman's battle with breast cancer." *Click*..."This season Murphy Brown faces breast cancer." *Click*...

OK, so it was Breast Cancer Awareness Month. I was aware already!

It did provide a lot of information though that might not have come to my attention at any other time. I might not have heard about the National Breast Cancer Alliance with its local chapter, devoted to advocacy for breast cancer legislation regarding research funding, insurance regulations, testing safety and procedures and other vital issues. This would be another organization for me to get involved with.

It seemed important to me to reach out and get involved in organizations like this. I could learn, and perhaps I could help someone else. I also talked to everyone I knew. Often a conversation with a friend or business associate would conclude with something like this:

"Is there anything I can do, Judy?"

"Yes, be sure that you and every woman you know has regular breast exams."

Even when talking with men, I would tell them to be sure their wife, mother, daughter, sister, aunt, were aware of the statistic that one woman in eight would be diagnosed with breast cancer every year.

My sister-in-law Theresa said she called for an appointment for a mammogram the week following my diagnosis.

My friend Linda asked, "What is your doctor's name? I need to make an appointment to get a mammogram. I've never had one."

I'm not certain how many breast exams and mammograms I may have been responsible for, but I hope it was a lot.

That is why I think it is so important to reach out and talk to everyone you know, not just about your cancer, but about their own health check-ups. Remember, I didn't feel sick. And it didn't feel like a distinctive "lump" that screamed breast cancer.

I told friends that if they encountered anything unusual in their breast not to accept these words from their doctor: "I don't think this is anything to be concerned about; we'll just keep an eye on it."

"Insist on a biopsy immediately," I told them, "and don't put it off out of fear of what you might find. The unknown is much more frightening!" Yeah, right, you can "keep an eye on it" and let it keep growing for a year like I did!

I stayed in touch with the two men, business associates and friends, who were diagnosed with different types of cancer at the same time I was. We talked frequently, keeping updated on each other's treatments and progress. With both Ed and Frank, I sort of formed one-on-one Cancer Club pals. And of course, I told both of them about K.B.

I told my friend Sandy in Seattle about K.B. and she couldn't stop laughing. I later got a Christmas card from her daughter, Kris, with this note: "I haven't even seen your bunny, but I love him anyway!"

One of the hardest things I had to do was talk to my nieces. "You girls be careful," I told them. "Be very aware; do self exams; get regular exams."

"Yeah, yeah, sure, Aunt Judy," was the look I got at first.

Until I continued, "Look, I feel guilty enough about this. I mean, until now, none of you had a family history of breast cancer. Now, thanks to me, you do."

Some legacy.

Somehow I had to let people know that I was maintaining my sense of humor through all of this too. I also had to let them know that I was doing OK, unless of course I was having a bad day and I would have to let them know that too.

Sometimes I didn't feel well from chemo or from lack of sleep. Sometimes I would get depressed when I washed my hair and clogged up the drain with all that had come out. I also got down when, half-way through chemo, the drugs seemed to be sending me through early menopause! *Great!* I thought. *I figured I'd have at least ten years before that showed up!* But through it all, I had to keep the humor going.

The Wellness Community understands the importance of humor and hosts an annual "JokeFest" for patients and their families. Everyone is a comedian and shares their favorite jokes in an uplifting and somewhat raucous evening.

I watched videotapes of recent reruns of the Flip Wilson show—which still sends me into hysterical laughter, as it did originally in the 1960's.

Comedy shows on TV were my mainstay. I avoided anything too serious, grim, heart-wrenching or sad. Supposedly a laugh that extends beyond fifteen or twenty seconds causes the body to release endorphins into the blood stream—these are the body's own "feel good" chemicals creating a natural and healthy "high".

I wrote our annual Christmas poem to go with our Christmas cards. I had been doing this for several years and friends said how much they enjoyed it. Instead of doing a typical "family newsletter" I always made mine fit the cadence of "The Night Before Christmas." While recounting our travels and what was happening in our family, it was usually amusing and somewhat tongue-in-cheek.

I managed to squeak one out that year, but it was the hardest one I'd ever written. I managed to find ways of referring to the year's cancer experience without dwelling on it. I had a few lines I was particularly proud of. It also made a huge positive impression on friends and family. Each year I entitle it, "Happy Holidays From Your Favorite Pair of Shorts!"

One friend wrote back: "What a delightful surprise to get your card and Christmas poem the other day! I don't think I would have had the fortitude or the discipline to sit down and create yet another sweet gift for my friends. You are indeed something special."

You be the judge:

Twas the month before Christmas when at breakfast my spouse
            Said, "You must write the poem!" and I started to grouse.
I shook my head slowly with the start of a tear,
            "I just really don't think I can write one this year."
"You can! You must!" he urged; he cajoled.
            "Everyone enjoys it and you can't leave them cold!"
Maybe he's right, I thought, smiling at him,
            The last fourth of the year was really all that was grim.
I started, "On Comet, On Cupid, On Prancer..."
            "OK," I stopped, "There's one rhyme for cancer."
The surgery went well and the chemo's not bad,
            And there were fun times before in this year that we had.
We started in January with the barefoot cruise,
            Just four friends and us to sail wherever we'd choose;

Rog, our chef, sustained us as we managed (surprise!)
       A 42-foot boat through the B.V.I.s!*
Monthly trips to Atlanta stayed first on our list,
       For two grandkids needed to be spoiled and kissed.
Steve & Becky & Spencer & Audrey are well,
       But still too far away, we're quite quick to tell.
Then most Mondays, Suzanne (in Cincinnati & nearby)
       Would come over and watch Melrose and laugh till we'd cry.
Business conventions brought travel (quite nice) —
       We LOVE the Big Easy—and hit Nawlins twice!
We lazed through July 4th on the isle of Nantucket
       You've all heard the limerick so I won't say…(forget it.)
We rode bikes and each ate a lobster a day,
       With a meeting first in Newport, all as gorgeous as they say.
Plus occasional trips to Baltimore and D.C.
       With our rented-out condo and friends there to see.
So it's been quite a year, from its highs to its lows;
       You really learn to appreciate what's right under your nose.
But the love and the prayers of our family and friends
       Give us strength and the healing power that sends.
So may your holidays be festive as ours will be
       While I'm putting a pink ribbon on top of our tree.
We send you our love and our hope and our cheer
       And wish you a healthy and happy New Year!

* British Virgin Islands

         *   *   *

On a day to day basis, I always tried to be honest in my response to the question, "How are you doing?"

Usually, the response would be: "Chemo's going well and I feel great!"

The person on the other end of this conversation would generally shake their head somewhat dubiously and say, "Well, you look great!"— as if they couldn't quite believe their eyes.

One of the women in my Cancer Club said that the response she usually got she found annoying at first, then would just shake her head and laugh about it eventually.

She said that she has always been in the habit of greeting people with a cheery, "Hi! How are you?"

After her cancer experience she said that others would always drop their head and their tone of voice and respond, "Oh, no, how are *you*?"

Sometimes though, I would run out of steam and just be amazingly tired. I would be honest about that too, telling my staff that I was going to lie down on the sofa in my office for a while or that I was just going to leave early. I figured there was no sense in dragging around, causing everyone to worry about me.

I went to a Christmas party that year and had labored over what to wear. I finally knocked everyone out by wearing a short dress with killer boots and rhinestone earrings. As people arrived, their immediate response with no trace of doubt in their voices was, "You look great!" I was not the picture of what they expected a cancer patient to look like.

When I learned of anyone, even an acquaintance, diagnosed with cancer or with a recent diagnosis in their family, I would reach out to them. The response was amazing when I would call and offer my support, based on experience. Not once did anyone seem to resent it or consider it an intrusion. It was as though I were throwing out a lifeline and they grabbed on eagerly. It's a funny thing, this camaraderie of cancer.

Chapter Eight

The Sounds of Silence

Every book I've read and every person I have talked with reports the same phenomenon: There is always at least one person, one friend or one family member, who cannot deal with the fact that you have cancer. With apologies to Simon and Garfunkel, I called this "The Sounds of Silence (S.O.S.)".

When I first heard about this, I thought, *Wow, that must be really hard. These people must have some serious mental problems to ignore someone with cancer! I'm glad no one I know would be like that.*"

Then, of course, it happened to me.

But the simple fact is that some people just find it too painful to deal with your pain. I've thought of any number of reasons for this, all of them plausible, all of them valid.

The person may have lost a loved one to cancer or some other disease, and cannot emotionally deal with it again right now.

The person may have a difficult time expressing his or her own emotions at your mortality—and consequently their own.

The person may never have encountered anything like this and have never had to express emotions verbally before.

The person may think they would be intruding or disturbing you if they called or dropped by, thinking maybe you'll be resting or not feel up to company or talking to anyone. Then this pattern just becomes a habit, too much time passes and the person feels awkward—and you just never hear from them.

The person may be so stunned at the news that they simply don't know what to say, so they say nothing, and subsequently do nothing—classic S.O.S.

At first I was so overwhelmed with the outpouring of love and support, flowers and cards, that I honestly thought that S.O.S. would not be a part of my cancer experience.

But of course, it was. Slowly, I came to realize the one or two people that I had not heard from. All the advice that I had heard or read said that you should make the first move, go ahead and call them if you feel like it. Let them know how you're doing and reassure them.

I couldn't do it. Others have said that they felt the same way, perhaps with a touch of anger. *If they don't care enough about me to pick up the phone and call or even send me a card, to heck with them!* That's not a very healing attitude for someone who needs all the positive strength they can muster to boost their immune system.

My answer to S.O.S. was to let it go. I told myself that anger wasn't healthy or loving. I allowed that this was really the other person's problem to deal with, not mine. They would come around in time, or there was not enough love there to begin with to sustain the relationship. I was sad and chagrined at first, but I learned to let go of the situation. Whatever happened, happened.

Then, over time, occasions may present themselves when you feel comfortable making that first overture.

A friend in my Cancer Club shared that she was very hurt and angry that she had not heard a peep from a friend of thirty years—who lived just four houses away. We suggested that she simply write a note in a Christmas card, inviting the friend to stop by sometime during the holidays.

Another reported that one of her closest friends simply vanished from her life shortly after her diagnosis. She simply never heard from her again.

Just remember that the person in your life who is stricken with S.O.S. is most probably thinking of you too. The S.O.S. may very well be their own distress signal, that they need help dealing with your illness, your pain, or with their own emotions. You can pray that they find help and strength or you can be the one to initiate it. It does not mean that they do not love you or do not care about you. The Sounds of Silence definitely speak louder than words.

In some cases you may be surprised to find that the Sounds of Silence are actually emanating from YOU. I have a couple of friends that I just couldn't call with the news. I couldn't handle the thought of dealing with *their* reaction. Some friends are simply too demanding, too needy. Where I felt that I had always been the one to do the giving in the friendship, I just didn't have the strength to keep giving in this situation. I prayed they would understand and not be too hurt, but for once I had to put my own well-being first.

I would not allow myself to feel guilty about this either. I was finding that cancer tends to free you from the "shoulds" and "ought to's" in life.

The main thing for you to do is concentrate on all the positives, and on all of those who are not silent.

I thought of the dear friends who had very valid reasons to shy away—but did not.

How hard this must have been for my friend Darla, who had been through many trying times in her own life recently. But she was constantly there for me.

Or my wonderful friend Carol, who had lost her mother, brother and uncle to cancer. Yet she could bravely come over a thousand miles to be with me during surgery.

Or one of my oldest and closest friends, Linda, whose mother had passed away earlier in the year. Yet there Linda was, at the hospital and at the house after I came home.

Roger's brother John and his wife Robin drove a hundred miles from Louisville with their daughter Lauren to visit me in the hospital and called constantly after I came home. John lost a kidney to cancer the year before and had given us quite a scare. Yet these loving family members were there for me.

My brother Joe and sister-in-law Teresa offered to come more than two hundred miles from Indiana to be with me during surgery, but I told them I'd rather they made the long trip after I got home and could spend more time visiting with them. So they came two weeks later, six days before my niece Mandy's wedding when Lord knows how much they had to do!

My older brother Bill and his wife Margge called frequently from Arkansas to check on me and offer their prayers and support.

One of my most precious keepsakes from this experience is an audio-tape that I dubbed off of our answering machine.

Roger, Carol and Larry and I had gone out to dinner the night before my first surgery. When we got home there were messages on the answering machine from my brother Joe and from our grandson Spencer. Spencer's message was the keeper.

"Hi, Nana," came that sweet little voice out of the machine. "I just wanted to say that I hope your surgery goes well and that I will say a pwayer (sic) for you. I love you."

Roger came into the bedroom after I had played it and found me standing there with tears streaming down my face.

"Honey, what's wrong?" he asked anxiously.

"Nothing," I muttered through my tears. "But you've all got to hear this."

So I called Carol and Larry in and hit the "play" button.

Then I went and got my portable tape recorder and immediately copied the message so I could keep it forever. Not quite five years of age, here was one young man who had no difficulty at all expressing his emotions, albeit prompted by his mom, I'm sure. He was old enough to understand that Nana was sick. He was old enough to understand that I needed him to send his love. I have a feeling that when he grows up, he will never be afflicted by S.O.S.

My most constant friend was totally silent, but his expression spoke volumes. There were days when K.B. seemed to be the most faithful and confident friend I had. If I didn't feel like talking to Roger or anyone else, I could always talk to K.B.

Some days I would look intently at him, wondering, *Where did this bizarre creature come from?*

Of course, I knew that I had conceived him and that Roger had created him. Yet he seemed so powerful, so in control, that I couldn't believe I made him up!

He reminded me that others might be silent too. He impressed upon me the basic truth that if I could accept his silence, I should be able to accept theirs as well.

When I meditated with him, I would envision this army of white bunnies, white blood cells, attacking and eating the cancer cells. I would see those white cells doubling, then doubling again. I kept repeating, "When there's more of us than there are cancer cells, we will win!"

I envisioned myself in the future, healthy and vibrant (with my longed-for flat stomach) sharing my story with other cancer patients.

I would envision myself twenty or more years in the future, older but healthy, sitting with Roger, at Spencer's wedding. Then at Audrey's.

Some days I would hold K.B. in front of me and talk to him like a drill sergeant with a new recruit.

"K.B., you've got to work harder! Multiply, you little sex fiend!"

Some days I would hold him and cry. "How did we wind up in this nightmare, K.B.? What are we going to do about it?"

He would stare back at me with unblinking eyes, teeth bared.

That is when I would hold him and squeeze his stomach and his head would flail back. It would seem that he was roaring, with those teeth really gnashing. He was truly a fighter—and so was I!

I would hold him and cry, "I love you, K.B. Whatever would I do without you?"

Then I was refocused on what we were going to do. We were going to fight hard and not give up or give in. We were going to beat this thing!

This kind of silence I could endure. It allowed me to hear my own heart.

Sidebar in this chapter:

S.O.S. and Things You "Hear" Later

Just a couple of weeks after my surgery, I had to miss my niece Mandy's wedding. I wasn't yet up and walking all that well and knew I could not endure a four-hour car ride to get there. It broke my heart. It was a major family event and I wouldn't be there. Her brother Blaine, whom I had not seen in ages and was stationed in Japan with the Marine Corps, was flying home to give her away. Nicol, Shanon and Annette, my other nieces, were all going to be part of the wedding.

I had written a funny poem to the tune of "The Beverly Hillbillies" that we were all going to sing at the reception, just for the fun of mortifying Mandy and welcoming her bridegroom into our loving, albeit dysfunctional, family. (She had made the mistake of mentioning to her mom that she had told her friends at work that her family was all a bunch of rednecks. *We'd show her!*)

In our family we are all a little bit nuts and very proud of it. How could I miss this? The wedding would be held in my hometown, in a church that Roger had designed. So many friends would be there whom I had not seen in years. Every time I thought about it, I cried.

I cried again the morning after the wedding when Mandy called as she and Chris were leaving for Las Vegas on their honeymoon. How sweet she was to call at such a hectic time and tell me that Roger and I were missed. She thanked me for the poem too and said it was "Quite the hit!" Again, you be the judge.

The Ballad for Mandy's Wedding Reception
(To the tune of "The Beverly Hillbillies")

Come and listen to the story
'Bout a gal named Mandy;
She's as sweet as a jar
Full of maple sugar candy;
We really love her —
She's a purty little miss;
Now she's gone off and married her a feller named Chris —
(Meng*, that is;
Handsome dude!)

Now Mandy went to work and was tellin' every friend:
"You can come to my weddin' but just ignore my kin;
"They're all a bunch of rednecks and
they're really kinda rude —
"They'll drink up all the likker and they'll eat up all the food!"
(Sloppy folks —
        Disgrace a pig!)

So we all promised Mandy
That we wouldn't make her blush;
Though we ain't got all our teeth,
We'd just go ahead and brush!
Mandy and Chris will be leavin' purty soon —
Goin' off to Vegas and we promised not to moon!
        (Honeymoon!!!

Married folks!)
Y'all come back now, ya hear?

Meng is Chris' last name.

I cried again at Christmas when I finally saw the photos of all that I had missed. I cried because I had felt that I was there that day, and as it turned out, everyone else felt that I was there too. They made sure of it.

At the reception, copies of my poem were placed on all the tables. My brother Joe and the whole family got up at the reception to sing the song, then lead the whole assembly in singing it again (several times). Before they began Joe told everyone, "This is a special song for Mandy and Chris written by my sister Judy. Aunt Judy couldn't be here today because she just had surgery for breast cancer and that's why all of us are wearing pink ribbons today. She's with us in spirit and we're with her."

I looked and there they all were: a pink ribbon on the wedding dress, pink ribbons on the bridesmaid dresses, pink ribbons on all the tuxedos, suits and special dresses.

They weren't all silent after all. Those pink ribbons spoke louder than words!

I looked at all my family gathered there for Christmas, kissed them all and thanked them. And we all cried some more, but at least we were all together then.

There were guests at that wedding, old friends, that I never heard from, but that was OK. I knew then that they had been thinking of me that day, sending me their positive thoughts and prayers, and that was really all that mattered.

Chapter Nine

Let Go and Let Others

One of the hardest parts of being ill is that you can't do what you always did before, at least for a temporary time period. It's an important part of healing to let go and let other people do things for us. It's also important to realize that OUR way isn't necessarily the right way or the only way and that in some cases "good enough" really is good enough.

Roger said I kept giving him directions on how to do things. He had always been great at pitching in around the house. He made ironing an art form. He loved to cook. But we usually did all these things as a team. If he cooked, I cleaned up. But now he had all his usual household chores—plus mine. After his gentle (if not so subtle) hint, I quit giving him my "helpful" directions on how to do the laundry, clean out the litter box, etc.

One woman in my Cancer Club said that nothing was done as well as she would have done it and that it was hard to accept that. Another said she was actually glad to be on a brief hiatus from ten years of volunteer work—let some other kid's mom volunteer for a change. Perhaps it was a coincidence, but I wondered if all this indicated more of a cancer "type" that all the women in my Cancer Club shared these same feelings. It seemed that we were a group of chronic over-achievers, if not downright perfectionists! Or it may just be that those of us who are used to getting things done are the type to seek out a support group to DO something about our cancer.

It may be very difficult at first, but it is so important to let people do things for you! If they didn't want to, they wouldn't offer. So sit back and be on the receiving end of things for a change. Perhaps these examples will give you (and your family and friends who read this) some ideas on what they can do for you.

Two elderly neighbor ladies were great about stopping by and dropping off food—from an entire dinner to soup to a loaf of banana bread. Again, I felt guilty at first. These wonderful women are older than me, with health problems of their own, yet here they were, waiting on me! (It also made me realize a need to be a more giving person myself when I got better.)

Our friends Carol and Larry who came back from Arizona to be with us during my surgery asked what they could do. I really couldn't think of anything specifically, but did mention that I was worried about Seka, our long-haired calico cat. She seemed to be losing weight and was listless. But on top of everything I was going through and all the doctor appointments and tests I was having, I just couldn't deal with finding a vet and having her checked out.

So Carol and Larry jumped on it. Two days after my surgery, they took her to a veterinary specialist who diagnosed her problem and referred us to a surgeon. This made it much simpler for Roger to then take the little furball in to have what turned out to be a benign (thank God!) tumor removed from her thyroid. It was bad enough that I had cancer, but I couldn't bear the thought of something happening to my cat too! (Jazmin, our other cat, seemed totally baffled by all that was going on.)

To me this was one of the greatest acts of friendship and love, though you may think that what they did was unusual. Carol and Larry understood, however, the importance of pets, as well as the value of me checking one item off on my list of things to worry about.

Yet another friend sent her hairdresser to the house the week after I got out of the hospital. "I just thought it was something I could do that would make you feel better," she said when she called to set it up. "I know what it's like when you've been in the hospital and since you can't move your left arm all that well right now, a 'do' might just perk you up."

She was right and I was thrilled at her thoughtfulness.

Another friend stopped by one day with some homemade chicken soup and one of the "Chicken Soup for the Soul" books. While we were visiting, a small family crisis arose and she quickly volunteered to take spare keys to rescue Suzanne who had just locked hers in her car.

My friends Linda and Darla took turns coming over to "babysit" me when I first got out of the hospital. It was difficult to get up and down without someone to lean on or help me and they were wonderful. Roger needed to get back to the office and couldn't be with me every second of every day.

So when Linda or Darla came over, we talked, watched videos, played backgammon or word games to pass the time. It's a wonderful lift to have friends stop by for a visit, but it's a real gift of love to spend a whole day entertaining a sick person! They both came to the hospital to see me too and Linda even spent a whole day there. She finally called home at supper time and her son Matt was worried, wondering where she was. After she explained she handed the phone to me. Linda had lived next door to us when Matt was born, so he was a pretty special kid to me, even if he was now a senior in high school.

"So," I joked with him. "You were worried about your mom and she didn't leave you a note where she was going?"

"Yeah," he laughed dryly. "It's a phase she's going through."

Under strict orders from Dr. Neale, I could not lift anything heavier than a gallon of milk—eight pounds was the max. Roger insisted that my purse weighed more than that and ordered me to get rid of the many "essential" items I thought I had to carry around.

When Thanksgiving rolled around two months after surgery, I faced a real dilemma. We went to Atlanta to see the grandkids for the first time since surgery. How could I possibly not pick up baby Audrey when she held those little arms up to Nana?

My oncologist Dr. Lower in her infinite wisdom warned me not to be too skittish around the kids. "You don't want them to think there's something wrong with them, which is the message little ones can get if they don't understand what's going on," she cautioned me.

Steve and Becky had talked to Spencer before our arrival and told him to be very careful about sitting on Nana's lap, because of the surgery. They warned him not to jump on me or rough-house like we usually did.

I quickly dispelled his (and their) worries by pulling him onto my lap. At first he was reluctant and said, "Mommy and Daddy said I can't sit on your lap because of your surgery."

"Don't worry about that," I reassured him, pulling him close. "Just don't lean on me too hard and we'll do just fine."

He relaxed and snuggled closer.

Audrey, at only seventeen months of age, was a little more difficult. She and I have been amazingly close. I even dreamed about her before she was born. When we had visited Labor Day Weekend, I had given her a bath and then prepared to give Spencer his bath. When Becky came to retrieve Audrey, she pulled away from Mommy, clinging to me. I don't know who was more shocked—me or Becky!

So when those little arms went up to me, it broke my heart not to be able to pick her up. I quickly worked out a system. Instead of picking her up, I would kneel on the floor and ease her onto my bended knee as she grabbed my neck. Then I would motion frantically for someone—any adult nearby—to pick her up and I would scurry to the nearest chair and have them set her on my lap. I'm sure she thought it was a confusing maneuver, but we both wound up with what we wanted. (OK, so I cheated a couple of times, but I didn't carry her far.)

Roger voiced what I was thinking—that it was our greatest Thanksgiving ever. I'll never forget Steve's prayer before our meal, surprised at first because Spencer usually had that honor. But Steve had some adult thoughts to express. He concluded with, "Thank you, Lord, that we can all be together and that Nana is doing so well after her surgery." Amen. My heart was full of love and I quickly wiped away a tear.

I also found that there are things that you can do for others during this time. Becky's sister Molly and her husband Todd were also with us for Thanksgiving. Todd's annual obligation is to be the photographer at Thanksgiving and take a family photo of Steve, Becky and the kids for them to send with their Christmas cards. This year's session did not go well. It had to be repeated a few hours later, when a visit to the one-hour photo service revealed no truly acceptable photo in the first batch.

Molly and I had done our best antics behind Todd during the first session, trying to get the kids to smile naturally. Our tricks were not going to work during the second session however.

"Todd," I asked, "Is your flash battery fully charged so you can take several shots in quick succession?"

"Sure," he nodded.

"OK, then get ready," I warned. Then I whipped off my wig and dropped it on Todd's head! (Todd is a Captain in the Marine Corps, so his military haircut made him look even more hilarious in my wig!)

The kids cracked up, and their Christmas photo that year will always be my absolute favorite.

My office staff was wonderful during this time as well, picking up the slack in my absence, but also continuing to do their usual duties. I knew I could count on them to keep all our activities and programs going and they came through. One staff member was elected to be the one to come up to the hospital to see me. They didn't want to all overwhelm me but wanted a first-hand report.

Since all my doctors' offices were nearby, I would usually insist that Roger stop by the office either before or after appointments when I got out of the hospital. The first time, just one week after surgery, everyone just came out to the curb to say "Hi." They also presented me with a thoughtful gift of a sleep shirt—with cats all over it. Our bookkeeper brought out checks for me to sign—which made me feel very useful. I was only out of the office about two weeks and I was eager to get back at it. The hardest part about lying around during healing and recovery—is the lying around. For an active person, this part can be boring and nerve-wracking. You have to teach yourself to relax and know that all those things will be waiting for you when you feel better.

Others in my Cancer Club often faced difficult decisions regarding their careers. I was fortunate that I was not in such a predicament with my job. My staff and board of directors were supportive, wanting me to do whatever it took to "get Judy well." I felt like I had the entire construction industry on my side. I received cards, flowers, phone calls and visits from so many of them which touched me deeply. I counted myself very fortunate to work for a group of people that I could also count as my friends.

One woman in my Cancer Club decided to step down from a key management position so that she could concentrate all her energies on her recovery during her treatment and healing process. Another was asked to step down from a high level job, but was offered a lesser position at the same pay.

What traumatic decisions these were and my hearts went out to these brave women! Though in different fields they had both worked all their lives to achieve success in their careers just as I had. Cancer does demand time from other obligations and duties. Sometimes difficult choices have to be made—or are made for you. Cancer demands that you set priorities—what is important to you and how do you want to spend your time? Through it all there is that nagging sense of loss of control—whether it is in the business world or at home. It is so difficult to let go of the responsibilities that have defined our lives before cancer, from work assignments to cooked meals to car pooling kids to even tending a sick cat.

It's emotionally draining to realize that your world has been turned upside down by cancer. It can be emotionally uplifting to realize that friends, neighbors, co-workers can and will do things for you, out of love and/or necessity. This can be a freeing time to reflect on your own priorities and what you really want to be when you "grow up." What do you really want to do with the rest of your life, after cancer? You can't move on to this new level until you let go of the life you knew before. So let others do those things you mastered in that old life, giving you time to master what your future will be.

I also had to let go and let K.B. do his job. Anyone who has ever gone through chemotherapy will understand how obsessed you become with your white blood count. K.B. and his friends had to be diligent in their assignment to keep reproducing, to keep my white count up. Before my third treatment I charged him with a specific assignment.

When I began chemo, my white count was at 6.8, with the normal range being somewhere between 4.6 and 10.2. Two weeks after my first treatment it had dropped to 4.3, but started coming back up the next week to 4.7 when I had my second treatment.

Because of the Christmas holidays, I had to shift my schedule, making my third treatment after four weeks instead of three. I figured K.B. could use that extra week to get that count back up. Every day I would hold him firmly and tell him to get to work. "When I get that report this week, I want to see a white count of at least 5. You can do it! Work! Work!"

Roger thought that an even more specific number would be appropriate and fixed on 5.2.

All that week I kept thinking to myself and to K.B., "Five…five point two…Make that white count match my height!"

When I went in for chemo I held K.B. tightly. "OK, K.B., this is your moment of truth. Let's see what you're made of." I just knew we'd make it.

As the nurse led Roger and me to an examining room, she handed us a copy of the blood report from the pinprick she had taken just minutes before. I stopped walking and stared in disbelief.

"You did it, K.B.!" I squealed, squeezing him and doing a little dance in the hallway, waving the report at Roger.

In the midst of my wild antics he couldn't focus on the computer printout and eagerly asked, "What is it? What is it?"

I looked at him triumphantly and declared, "Nine point eight! Oh, we of little faith were shooting a bit too low for K.B.!"

Killer Bunnies RULE! I thought, shaking my head happily.

Chapter Ten

You Won't Be Glad You Had Cancer But...

The week after I got home from the hospital, I received a phone call from my friend John whom I had worked with in D.C. John and I had actually teamed up on industry-wide projects before I was hired by the same association where he worked.

Shortly after we met, John's wife Helen experienced much of what I was now going through during her own battle with breast cancer. Helen has been cancer-free for many years now, but I knew how hard this phone call had to be for John, bringing up all the memories. That's probably why it meant so much and why he suggested that I give Helen a call.

I will never forget the words of this sweet Tennessee belle to me.

"Judy, I don't really know how to say this, but in time you'll under-stand what I'm getting at. You won't be glad that you had cancer. But in some strange way, you will be very thankful for the experience. It will change your whole life, your priorities, and your perspective. You will never be the same."

I know that Helen was right. All of those things have happened to me already.

Relationships grow stronger. Little things don't bother me any more. I'm more open about my feelings when things do bother me. I let people know and get it off my chest, in a tactful way. I don't feel like I have to be SuperWoman and make everything right for everyone else. I know that I have to take care of me first, before I can possibly do anything for anyone else—whether it's in my work, my family, my friendships, or any outreach that I do for others.

My Cancer Club ended after its programmed twelve-week sessions, but we still get together occasionally for lunch. We developed deep friendships and we want to keep in touch and up to date on how everyone in the group is doing.

When we first started talking about getting together, we discussed whether we would join one of the other ongoing support groups at The Wellness Community. Most of us were hesitant at first. I mean, we were getting well! We didn't want to be around a bunch of people in worse shape than us, or who were experiencing a recurrence of their cancer. We were determined that we wouldn't be one of those statistics.

Before the final session ended, Chris, our facilitator, interjected this bombshell. "What if one of you does have a recurrence?"

There was silence in the room. Then all at once several people burst out with, "Well, then we're not going to tell that person where we're meeting for lunch!"

We all broke up into helpless laughter.

Because we all knew that it wasn't true.

If it were one of our own, we would be there for her.

It was a sobering thought nonetheless. We all knew that we would never in our lives be free of that fear. The statistics are frightening—that 50% of the people who have cancer won't make it. That is discouraging and depressing and I even hesitate to write that here, but you'll read it elsewhere. The main thing is to be determined to be in that other 50%.

One woman in our Cancer Club said that when she heard or read of someone dying of cancer, she wasn't cold-heartedly glad they died— but figured it increased her chances. There was another one for the OTHER 50%!

You know that you're going to spend the rest of your life waiting for the other shoe to drop. Will you feel safe after being cancer-free for five years, or seven years, or twenty years? Probably not. You simply have to be determined not to let that fear ruin your life or turn you into a hypochondriac. *Uh, oh, I have a pain in my side. Do I have liver cancer? My legs ache all the time. Do I have bone cancer?* Every lump or knot becomes a nightmare.

You have to dismiss those negative thoughts. What will I do if I have a recurrence? Well, K.B. and I will just have to deal with that if and when the time comes.

None of us ever knows how much time we have anyway in any circumstance. This cancer experience just sharpens the focus; it speeds up the time line. What happens if the cancer comes back? Well, what if I get hit by a bus tomorrow? Either way, there are no guarantees.

Many friends in my Cancer Club reported a sense of not putting off things they had dreamed of doing. One took a trip to France with her family after her surgery but before chemo started. Another cashed in some retirement funds and went with her husband on their lifetime dream trip of a cruise to Alaska.

Others reported that they did put off things that no longer seemed so important, from day to day chores they used to obsess about to longer term obligations that fell into the "ought to" or "should" category.

I actually found myself to be a little less patient than before. *Hurry up! Out of my way!* I would think. *I don't know how much time I have.* Eventually, I found a balance.

Roger and I participate in the Susan G. Komen Race for the Cure and the American Cancer Society's "Making Strides for Breast Cancer"— as walkers, not runners. I am very proud of my pink shirt and pink "survivor's" hat. I don't feel alone. There are just so many of us. It is an emotional experience and I feel so lucky to be there, lucky to be alive.

I will continue living life by the rules given me by Dr. Lower during chemo. If you feel like doing it, do it. If you don't feel like doing it, don't.

If it looks or sounds good, go ahead and eat or drink it. With moderation and common sense in mind, those are pretty good rules for anyone, any day of the week, cancer or no cancer.

When my hair thinned during chemo, I started wearing my wig. That was a very freeing experience. Most people didn't even notice. They just thought I'd gotten a new hairstyle, and a very flattering one at that. (Yeah, right, my hair might ever look that good every day.)

The first time I wore it to Atlanta to see the kids, Steve didn't even realize it was a wig. He commented to Becky, "Judy's new hairstyle is really nice."

"Yeah," Becky said. "It looks really natural."

"Uh, what do you mean, it looks natural?" came back Mr. Clueless.

"Steve, it's her cranial prosthesis! It's a wig!" Becky laughed.

Pretty cool, huh? Plus everyone was jealous and wanted to get one too. It's definitely the all-time cure for bad hair days. When our grandson was being potty trained he insisted on wearing "easy" pants, with elastic waists and no buttons or zippers. The wig was "easy" hair. Learning to live with these little "sidebars" of the cancer experience were part of my education too.

Figuring out how to dress was another challenge. Because of the abdominal incision for my breast reconstruction, my stomach was incredibly sensitive, swollen and painful for many, many months. This meant that I could not wear anything around my waist. No slacks, no pants, no leggings, no sweat suits, no skirts.

I was able to manage pretty well with my work wardrobe by rotating a number of jackets with several solid color dresses. However, casual clothes were a real challenge! Jumpers were about the only option.

Roger and Suzanne shopped for me endlessly. They bought me a denim jumper and several corduroy ones. Roger bought me some flat shoes and some docksider loafers. The fact that these shoes weren't in my closet before tells you pretty much how I usually dressed: Leggings and a tee-shirt or sweatshirt, usually bedecked with sparklies or glitter. (Steve asked me once if I even owned a plain shirt and of course, I didn't. Roger said that I was like a crow, immediately attracted to anything shiny.)

So this "new look" in my style of dressing took some getting used to. When Victoria, Dazy and Bambi came to visit from D.C. they would collapse into gales of laughter each morning when I emerged from the bedroom in one of my new ensembles.

Roger just shook his head. "You look like someone who should be named 'MariLu' or something. It's just such a wholesome, down-to-earth look!"

It was a look that definitely was NOT me and I hated it.

And the nickname "MariLu" stuck.

Shortly after his fifth birthday, our grandson Spencer asked me, "Nana, why does everyone call you MariLu?"

"Look at me," I said to him. "Does this look like something Nana would usually be wearing?"

(I was in my red velveteen Christmas jumper.)

He shook his little head immediately and said, "No," drawing the word out into several emphatic syllables.

"Well, honey," I explained, "Nana has to wear these clothes because of her surgery and they just look like something that someone named MariLu would wear."

It's amazing but it seemed that even one so young could grasp this concept of style.

I was so excited when we went to visit Carol and Larry in Arizona over New Year's and I bought a pair of black pants! OK, so they were really a jumpsuit type affair with a short bib in front and suspender type straps. But they were pants!

I had bought a fleecy top to wear with them, but my friend Carol came up with the ingenious idea that I could wear any of my bulky tops and sweaters OVER the straps—and then it just looked like a regular pair of pants.

I really was learning to find joy in the little things in life!

We have a really scary photograph that we keep to look at from time to time. Roger had it in a frame on his desk, but brought it home one day and said, "I can't look at this every day. It just freaks me out."

He had taken the photograph of me over the previous Fourth of July when we were in Nantucket —prior to my diagnosis. I was standing in front of a typical gray clapboard Nantucket house with pink flowers blooming wildly in front of it. Although it was a bright, sunny day, somehow I was standing where I cast a shadow on the front of my body—except where one patch of sunlight shone through in a full circle—surrounding my left breast. The circle of light lay almost exactly where my incision was later to be. When we got the photos back, we noticed it but didn't really think anything of it—until later.

No one who looked at the photo could figure out where that circle of light came from.

"Plus," Roger would add. "Look at your face. You're not smiling; you don't look happy."

Yet I knew that I was then. We were having a wonderful time, riding bikes, eating lobster and just taking it easy. How could Kodak have so accurately foretold my future? It's a sobering thought, but also a constant reminder that we cannot know what the next day, or in this case, the next month will bring.

Suzanne had been to a psychic in June just for fun. This woman had asked her, "Do you know anyone with breast cancer?"

Suzanne admitted that she didn't.

The psychic shook her head. "I see someone very close to you wearing a pink ribbon."

Suz told her roommate and some friends about it, but didn't mention it to us until later.

Oddly enough, over time both our cats even developed a special relationship with K.B.— but only when they were sick. Most of the time they ignored him like any other toy around the house. But when one of them was sick, she would go lie down next to K.B. or on his lap.

Sometimes they would meow at him or do that nursing or kneading motion with their feet that cats do. It was eerie, but it seemed that they were communicating, "Hey, Rabbit, I'm not feeling so good either and could use your help."

What do these strange things mean? I believe that they are examples from life that we cannot explain. If these occurrences can't be explained, then who is to say that my Killer Bunny has to have some logical explanation?

Looking back it seemed somehow poignant that I was diagnosed with cancer the same week that Princess Diana and Mother Theresa died. I don't count myself in their league by any means, but it just seemed to me that it was most definitely not a good week for women anywhere in the world, no matter who we were. Those two supreme role models also brought home to me the uncertainty of life and the value of making the most of each day—of making a difference in how we touch the lives of others, in what we accomplish.

There were difficult times when coping seemed impossible. The last three chemo sessions were rough. I was sicker; the anti-nausea drugs seemed to quit working as well; I was tired all the time.

My second surgery, for the rest of my reconstruction, went well but actually seemed more stressful than the first, more extensive operation. I didn't bounce back as quickly and took a longer time recovering. I realized that my body was weakened from all the chemo and that I had less stamina than the first time.

It seemed to take months to really start feeling better. My old energy and zip were a long time in returning. It got discouraging at times. I was sick and tired of feeling sick and tired. I finally realized what a long, hard road I have traveled.

Helen's words keep coming back. I'm not glad in any way that I had cancer. But the new me is wiser, surer, more in control of the things that I can control. I am thankful for a deeper sense of myself and the world around me. I listen better, to my heart and to others.

As a result of my fight with breast cancer, I know there are some marvelous people in the medical profession. I know how much the people who love me really do love me. I know that I can call on the power of my own body, mind and spirit to heal, to overcome illness, to defy negativity, to live life with a focus on meaningfulness and quality.

I have a certain rabbit with scary teeth and a take-charge attitude to thank for it. K.B., you are truly my hero.

About the Author

JUDITH TROTTER SHORT is a Certified Association Executive (CAE) and the Executive Director of Allied Construction Industries, a commercial construction trade association in Cincinnati, Ohio. A native of Indiana, she and her architect husband Roger enjoy traveling, cooking and spending time with their grandchildren, Spencer and Audrey.

Start your own Journal: